The Big
FIVE

The Big
FIVE

*Five Simple Things You Can Do
to Live a Longer, Healthier Life*

Dr. Sanjiv Chopra
with David Fisher

THOMAS DUNNE BOOKS
St. Martin's Press
New York

THOMAS DUNNE BOOKS.
An imprint of St. Martin's Press.

www.thomasdunnebooks.com
www.stmartins.com

Portions of this book have appeared in *Live Better, Live Longer* (2012)
and *Doctor Chopra Says* (2010).

The Library of Congress Cataloging-in-Publication Data is available
upon request.

ISBN 978-1-250-06533-9 (hardcover)
ISBN 978-1-4668-7213-4 (e-book)

Our books may be purchased in bulk for promotional, educational,
or business use. Please contact your local bookseller or the Macmillan
Corporate and Premium Sales Department at 1-800-221-7945, extension
5442, or by e-mail at MacmillanSpecialMarkets@macmillan.com.

First Edition: May 2016

10 9 8 7 6 5 4 3 2 1

CONTENTS

I dedicate this book to my granddaughters, Aanya and Mira, who are the wellspring of happiness and joy in my life and inspire me to live in harmony and with abundance.

INTRODUCTION

I have been a physician for more than four decades. For me, the profession of medicine has been more than a job or a career. It has been a calling. I love my work and find purpose and meaning in taking care of patients, starting by taking a detailed and thorough history and doing a skilled examination and formulating a diagnosis and treatment plan. It has been a privilege to be trusted to do so. I have also taught medicine not only throughout the United States but also in scores of countries abroad.

When I entered the profession, the art and practice of medicine was much simpler. In the last four decades, medicine has changed drastically and dramatically. We have witnessed the emergence of a modern pestilence—HIV/AIDS—from the first cases reported in 1981 to the toll of 39 million deaths worldwide by 2013. The diagnosis of AIDS back in the seventies was a death sentence. Now patients take one pill once a day and can live a full and healthy life. An example of this is the basketball legend Magic Johnson. He announced he had tested positive for HIV in 1991, and about a quarter century later he is still thriving.

Medicine has witnessed many triumphs, including the development of effective vaccines. The hepatitis B virus afflicts 400 million people worldwide. It can lead to cirrhosis, liver failure, and primary cancer of the liver, which is the third leading cause of cancer mortality worldwide. The hepatitis B vaccine is in a sense the first anticancer vaccine. Two decades of universal childhood vaccination in Taiwan led to a 75 percent reduction in childhood primary liver cancer mortality.

As we triumph, we also face new tragedies. Ebola is not a new disease, but the recent outbreak in West Africa has instilled deep fear in millions of people worldwide. Vaccine trials are in progress, and I am confident that in the near future a very safe and effective vaccine will be available for large-scale use.

Our understanding of many cancers, coronary heart disease, obesity, diabetes, Alzheimer's dementia, and other chronic disorders continues to advance at a remarkable pace. Some of the landmark discoveries and treatments have emerged from concerted and brilliant scientific investigations. Other major discoveries have occurred through the magic of serendipity. The word "serendipity" is derived from a story about the three princes of Serendip, who were "always making discoveries, by accidents and sagacity, of things which they were not in quest of." Examples include the discovery of penicillin and the bacteria H. pylori.

The best scientific studies are randomized, double-blind, placebo-controlled trials. The results can be trusted, and often these studies are published in the most prestigious medical journals. However, great insights can also be gleaned from large-scale, well-conducted, epidemiological studies. Epidemiology is the science that studies the patterns—incidents, distribution—and causes of health and disease in defined populations. Well-conducted studies identify risk factors for—sometimes even clues to the cause of—a major disease. They can lead to policy decisions, which, when enforced, can positively impact the health of large segments of the population.

One of the best-known epidemiological studies is the Framingham Heart Study, which began in 1948. Five thousand two hundred and nine adult subjects between the ages of thirty and sixty-two were recruited from Framingham, Massachusetts; the study now includes a third generation of participants. This longitudinal study has shed important light on heart disease, including the effect of smoking cigarettes, diet, exercise, obesity, and commonly used medicines, such as aspirin, on health and disease. Over a thousand scientific medical papers have been published from the knowledge obtained from this groundbreaking study.

Medicine continues to fascinate and dazzle me, from the promise of high-tech, glitzy innovations like stem cells and regenerative medicine to behaviors or habits that could be adopted by millions, even billions, of individuals for dramatic and long-lasting benefit.

In this book, I explore and explain the evidence regarding the incredible health benefits of coffee, vitamin D, exercise, meditation, and nuts. The evidence is conclusive. There is no doubt in my mind that drinking coffee, maintaining high but normal levels of vitamin D, exercising regularly, taking a few minutes each day to meditate, and eating a handful of nuts is very good for you. Of course, one or more of these things on occasion can be problematic. Some people have serious nut allergies; for others, drinking more than three or four cups of coffee a day can lead to insomnia and tremors.

But for the overwhelming majority of people, ensuring that these five common behaviors are part of one's daily routine can go a really long way toward promoting and maintaining good health and perhaps extending life.

The impact of these five modalities on health—coffee, vitamin D, exercise, meditation, and nuts—has been studied for decades. As I show in this book, numerous well-crafted studies involving many thousands of people have shown how we can accrue great benefits from these five simple lifestyles changes. There are no theories involved; this is real-world data showing what happens when you take certain actions. There is also no attempt to explain or even understand why this is true—it just is. The conclusions are only as good as the quality of the data and the researchers, so I have not included small studies or studies sponsored by the purveyors of coffee and nuts or those selling vitamin D. This has allowed me to say quite categorically that people who drink coffee, exercise, maintain sufficient vitamin D levels, meditate regularly, and eat nuts show proven benefits over people who don't. I often advise patients and friends to heed the following advice. On a nice sunny day, take a short, brisk walk to your favorite java shop. Enjoy the coffee, and if you're going to have a bite to eat, you might as well partake of a handful of nuts. You have now exercised, manufactured some vitamin D from the sun, and had coffee and nuts. It is that simple!

I want to mention that these are not the only behaviors that are good for you. There is also substantial, emerging evidence that a Mediterranean diet can also be very good for you. In a recent, large study published in the *British Medical Journal*, greater adherence to a Mediterranean diet was associated with longer telomeres. This study is fascinating, and it is very likely that in the not-too-distant future we will see many more scientific studies addressing telomeres and longevity.

There are also some interesting observational studies that conclude that expressing gratitude on a regular basis can lead to individuals feeling happy and perhaps living longer.

Obviously, you need to be wise about incorporating these five things into your lifestyle. Get advice from experts: before beginning a regular exercise program speak with a trainer and find out what works best for you and what your limitations are. Listen to your body after drinking that additional cup of coffee and see how it affects the rhythms of your day and night. See a doctor to determine if you are deficient in vitamin D and therefore should be taking a supplement. Make sure you have no nut allergies before dipping into a tray of nuts.

But if you really are searching for easy and inexpensive ways to support and maintain good health, these five behaviors should become part of your daily lifestyle.

I trust you will find the information in this book helpful. Heed the advice and live a healthier and longer life. I wish you and your family and friends the greatest of treasures, the gift of perfect health and many more years together.

W*orldwide, an estimated
2.25 billion cups of coffee
are consumed every day.*

I

COFFEE—
A CUP OF HEALTH

Americans love coffee. We drink about 400 million cups of coffee a day, making us the leading coffee-consuming nation in the world. An estimated 83 percent of American adults drink coffee. The average cup of coffee is nine ounces, and we drink about three cups every day. American coffee drinkers spend an average of $1,100 a year on coffee. Coffee is considered the ultimate energy drink. Most people drink it in the morning to get them going and in the afternoon to give them the necessary pick-up-up-up-up. "In Seattle," according to Amazon founder and CEO Jeff Bezos, "you haven't had enough coffee until you can thread a sewing machine while it's running."

Americans also drink it because we love its taste: about a third of all the coffee we buy is considered gourmet coffee, meaning it is espresso-based or otherwise a specialty drink.

We're not the only people who love coffee. Worldwide, an estimated 2.25 billion cups of coffee are consumed every day. Mostly we drink coffee because we love its taste and because it provides an instant energy boost. Former late-night host David Lettermen once admitted, "If it wasn't for coffee, I'd have no identifiable personality whatsoever."

With the meteoric rise of Starbucks and America's estimated 25,000 other coffee shops, the availability of various special preparations and blends of coffee, and the ease of one-cup coffeemakers, the once-bland world of coffee has been transformed into one of the fastest-growing food and beverage industries in the county. Business has discovered that coffee is indeed the multi-billion-dollar bean. Few people look forward to their daily stop at the local coffee shop more than I do. In addition to getting my coffee, I'm going to meet friends there, and we'll sit together for a few minutes enjoying our coffee and the joy of companionship.

But few people drink it for the most important reason: Coffee is really good for you. I make that statement as a physician and liver specialist. In fact, coffee actually may well be the healthiest beverage you can drink. Many people don't believe that. When I make that statement they sometimes look at me like I've told the beginning of a joke and they are waiting for the punch line. Often when I'm giving a lecture on a liver disorder, I will ask everyone in the audience who drinks at least two cups of coffee to raise their hands. Most hands, both of men and women, go up. "Good," I tell them, then ask, "How many of you drink at least four cups a day?" Fewer hands are raised, and I notice that people look around the room nervously to see who is drinking that much coffee. Finally I ask my audience, "How many of you average six or more cups of coffee a day?" In response there is always some sort of nervous laughter and then a few brave people gingerly raise their hands, as though they were doing something wrong. That's when I say to the audience, "You know what? It's good for you! You're really doing yourself a big favor."

In fact, instead of believing coffee is good for you, most

people believe it can be harmful. In the past drinking too much coffee supposedly had been linked to a variety of health problems including heart attacks, birth defects, pancreatic cancer, osteoporosis, weight gain, hypertension, and miscarriage. We do know that in some instances coffee can cause insomnia, tremors, raise blood pressure a tad, and worsen heartburn, and it certainly increases urination. For those reasons people usually limit the amount of coffee they drink and often decide that for health reasons they shouldn't have that extra cup of coffee they are craving. I often hear this common refrain: "Dr. Chopra, I used to drink two cups of coffee a day. Now I hardly drink it. Isn't caffeine bad for you?"

The evidence that they are misinformed is overwhelming, and more of it is being reported practically every day. While many people read those stories, they still don't believe them. Few people consider coffee a health drink. In fact, most people don't even know how effective coffee appears to be in preventing a variety of very serious illnesses, or, when they learn the facts, they remain quite dubious. They ask incredulously, "You're saying coffee is probably better for me than tea? Coffee really can reduce the risk of developing a number of common cancers? It can decrease the risk of developing gallstones and tooth decay? It decreases the risk of developing cirrhosis of the liver? It can even decrease the risk of developing dementia? Dr. Chopra, are you nuts?"

I have become a true advocate of the health benefits of coffee, so much so that many of my medical colleagues are amused by my passion for coffee. For years I spent four weeks attending on the in-patient hepatology service at Beth Israel Deaconess Medical Center, a major teaching affiliate of Harvard Medical School. To satisfy my own curiosity I instructed the students, interns, residents, and fellows to ask all the patients admitted with severe liver disease one additional question: How much coffee do you drink? The answer I always got was that none of our patients with severe liver disease regularly drank coffee. It's quite uncanny and quite remarkable how consistent this answer had been, week after week, for years. But a couple of years ago, as I was about to start teaching rounds, a resident approached me smiling broadly and said, "Dr. Chopra, we finally have a patient on our liver service who drinks four cups of coffee every day!"

Oh, well, that caught my attention. I said, "Tell me more about him."

The resident responded, "He's a fifty-three-year-old patient who was admitted yesterday with severe cellulitis."

I told the house staff, "When we go and see him at rounds, I will take my own history. He may well be the exception to the rule. The studies are epidemiological and may not be iron-clad, even though there are some reasonable mechanistic explanations."

When I met this patient I took a detailed history. In addition to the questions about alcohol and over-the-counter medications, I said to him, "Please tell me about tea and coffee. Do you drink any?"

"I don't drink tea at all," he said, shaking his head. "But I love coffee."

I asked him if he drank regular or decaf, since most studies had shown that it is regular coffee that confers major protection against liver disease.

"Only regular," he said, smiling, "If you're going to drink coffee you might as well drink the real thing."

I asked him how many cups of coffee he drank every day.

"At least four," he said, "sometimes more."

"What size?" I inquired.

He pointed to a large paper cup on his bedside table and said, "That size."

I asked one final question, "How long have you been drinking regular coffee?"

And matter-of-factly he responded, "Ever since my liver transplant." He then turned to me and asked, "Should I stop? Is it bad for me?"

"No, it's not," I said, repressing a laugh. "Keep drinking it, it's very good for you.

No wonder coffee hadn't prevented his disease. I asked him, "Did someone tell you to drink coffee after your transplant?"

He shook his head again. "It's really strange. I never used to like coffee, but after my transplant I suddenly had this incredible craving for coffee!" The facts are indisputable; coffee appears to offer a great variety of benefits, including substantial protection against liver cirrhosis, type 2 diabetes, heart disease, Parkinson's disease, cognitive decline and dementia, gallstones, tooth decay, and a host of common cancers, including prostate, colon, endometrial, and skin cancer. There also is a lower rate of suicide among coffee drinkers.

Incredible as it may seem, coffee also appears to make you smarter, can improve physical performance—major league baseball players may drink as many as six cups of coffee during a game to increase focus and response time—and even helps burn fat. It can be used to treat headaches, and, contrary to conventional wisdom, it appears to lower the risk of being hospitalized for arrhythmia.

But perhaps the single most startling conclusion that has

Coffee drinkers have
a lower risk of developing cirrhosis,
cancer of the liver,
and type 2 diabetes.

emerged from the more than 19,000 studies concerning the impact of coffee on health is that people who drink a lot of coffee appear to live longer than people who drink little or no coffee. That's an incredible statement, but there are several good studies that support it. A National Institutes of Health study published in the *New England Journal of Medicine* in 2012 analyzed data collected from 400,000 participants over a fourteen-year period and concluded that the overall mortality rate for people who drank between two and six cups of coffee a day was about 10 percent lower for men and about 15 percent lower for women. The study found that the more coffee participants drank, the more they cut their risk of death, with the greatest benefit seen in people who enjoyed four or five cups. Interestingly, women benefitted slightly more than men.

A Johns Hopkins Bloomberg School of Public Health review of twenty-one studies conducted between 1966 and 2013 that included almost a million participants concluded that people who drank as many as four cups of coffee daily reduced mortality by 16 percent.

There is one caveat though: Studies also show that coffee consumption often is linked with known health risks (e.g., coffee drinkers tend to smoke), which tends to skew the results.

Considering the myriad of potential health benefits to be gained from drinking coffee, it is somewhat surprising how little most Americans know about them. I am also surprised that an overwhelming number of physicians are not aware of the many benefits of coffee. If a patient says to his primary care physician, "I heard coffee has lots of health benefits," the response they often hear is, "These studies come and go.

Coffee drinkers,
both men and women,
have lower total and
cause-specific mortality
compared to those who
do not drink coffee.

Everything in moderation is okay." In reality, this is inaccurate. Scores and scores of well-conducted studies have been published in prestigious, peer-reviewed medical journals. There appears to be a dose-dependent effect—in other words, the more coffee an individual consumes on a daily basis, the greater the benefit or the risk reduction in many of the common medical ailments mentioned above.

While many people can rhapsodize for hours about the nuances of wines, the craft of creating beers, and the history and variations of teas, few people know much about coffee beyond how they order it each morning. But coffee has a rich and bold history and has helped shaped the world as much as any other substance.

Coffee does grow on trees. It is a very hearty plant that can grow in a great variety of conditions, which is why it is such an important economic crop. It is grown around the world. It takes three or four years for a coffee tree to bear fruit. That fruit, the coffee cherry, actually is a bright, deep red color. Rather than a bean, it is a seed, and if it is planted rather than processed it will grow into a tree. Most often these cherries are picked by hand, and in most countries there is a single annual harvest. It takes about two thousand cherries to produce one pound of roasted coffee. After the coffee is dried it is prepared for export, which can be done several different ways. An estimated seven million tons of this "green coffee," as it is now called, are shipped each year. This green coffee is finally roasted at about 550° into the aromatic brown beans that most of us recognize as coffee, then sold to the consumer while still fresh.

The legend is that the virtues of coffee were first discovered in the ninth century by a shepherd named Kaldi, who observed while tending his goats in the Ethiopian highlands that his flock became unusually active after eating the red berries from certain trees. Supposedly he told the abbot of the local monastery about this curious discovery. According to this story the abbot frowned upon this magical power and angrily threw the berries into the fire. The enticing aroma that arose from the burning beans attracted other residents of the monastery. These roasted beans were brewed into a drink and the monks discovered that it kept them awake and alert throughout the long hours of evening prayer. They shared this knowledge with other monks, and slowly stories about the powers of these red berries to create a vibrant consciousness began spreading throughout the world.

Other legends attribute the discovery of coffee to a Yeminite Sufi mystic who noticed, during his travels through Ethiopia, that birds feasting on these red berries seemed more energetic, and when he chewed the berry he enjoyed a similar response. While the truth will never be known, it is generally accepted that the properties of the coffee bean were discovered in Ethiopia and exported to Yemen. For hundreds of years coffee remained popular throughout the Islamic world. By the sixteenth century it had spread throughout the Middle East. The word "coffee," in fact, can be traced to the Arabic *qahwa,* a slang term meaning "wine of the bean." Turks translated that to be *kahve,* which the Dutch called *koffie* and which entered the English language as "coffee" in 1582.

In many places this *qahwa* was greeted with suspicion. What kind of strange brew causes such disruptions of the spirit? In 1511 imams in Mecca banned its use, but that ban was overturned a decade later by the Ottoman Turkish sultan. In 1532 it was outlawed in Cairo, and coffee storehouses were reduced to rubble. As it turned out though, it wasn't only Muslim clerics who tried to prevent the spread of this powerful and seemingly dangerous stimulant.

It was the globe-traveling merchants of Venice who introduced coffee to Europe, where it became known as "the Muslim drink." It created quite a . . . stir. The possible medicinal attributes of coffee were first noted in 1583, when German physician Leonhard Rauwolf, after returning from an exploration of the Near East, described "[a] beverage as black as ink, useful against numerous illnesses, particularly those of the stomach. . . . It is composed of water and the fruit from a bush called bunnu." Almost instantly there was a debate within the Catholic Church as to whether it would be permitted or banned; there is considerable dispute as to precisely which church leader eventually made the decision. Some credit Pope Clement VIII, while others believe it was Pope Vincent III, but the story goes that the pope demanded to taste it before rendering his decision and that, after doing so, rather than banning it he proclaimed, "Why, this Satan's drink is so delicious that it would be a pity to let the infidels have exclusive use of it. We shall cheat Satan by baptizing it."

At that time nations often tried to control the market for certain goods. While the Dutch attempts to prevent other nations from growing tulips is well known, there were similar efforts by coffee-growing regions to prevent the spread of the coffee tree. Nations guarded their coffee trees. In 1670 a smuggler strapped seven beans from Yemen onto his chest and carried them to India. When French King Louis XIV turned down a request for coffee tree clippings from a young naval officer from the colony of Martinique, that officer stole them and hid them aboard his ship. His voyage home was perilous, the ship was becalmed and the crew and passengers went without water for days—so he shared his precious allotment of these seeds. They survived the journey, and within half a century 18 million trees had been planted on Martinique and the coffee trade became a thriving industry.

Brazil grew to become the world's largest coffee exporter after dispatching a colonel to French Guiana purportedly to mediate a border dispute. In fact, he won the affections of the governor's wife, who handed him a bouquet of flowers at his farewell dinner—with coffee seeds hidden in the bouquet.

Among the prizes of war won by Austria after defeating the Turkish army in a 1683 battle were sacks of coffee beans. The Austrians created their own blend of coffee to be served with a cake called *kipfel*, which was shaped to resemble the crescent moon on the flag of the defeated Turkish army—and eventually became known by its French name, the croissant.

Proving that history repeats itself, for centuries most coffee was consumed in coffeehouses—historic versions of Starbucks—which served as centers of social and political activity. The first known coffeehouse opened in Istanbul in 1471. Europe's first coffeehouse opened its doors in Italy in 1645. In these "penny universities," as they became known in England because the cost of a cup was one penny, people could listen to music, play chess, watch performers, conduct business, and debate the issues of the day. Relationships that changed history were conducted in those meeting places; for example Lloyd's of London grew out of Lloyd's Coffee House. In some nations the political and religious discussions that became commonplace made governments wary, fearing rebellion was being plotted. England's Charles II tried to close down the estimated three thousand coffeehouses in that nation in December 1675, issuing a proclamation that read, in part, "Whereas it is most apparent that the multitude of Coffee Houses of late years set up and kept within this kingdom . . . and the great resort of idle and disaffected person to them, have produced very evil and dangerous effects . . . (and that) in such houses divers, false, malitious, and scandalous reports are devised and spread abroad to the . . . Disturbance of the Peace and Quiet of the Realm . . . said Coffee Houses be (for the future) put down and surpressed. . . ." Two weeks later, after widespread protests, the ban was rescinded.

Eventually coffeehouses became so respectable that Johann Sebastian Bach conducted an ensemble at the Café Zimmerman in Leipzig, Germany, for which he composed his *Coffee Cantata* in 1734: "Oh! How sweet coffee does taste, lovelier than a thousand kisses, sweeter than Muscatel wine. Coffee, coffee, I've got to have it, and if someone wants to pamper me, Oh, just give me a cup of coffee!"

In America, the tradition of the morning cup of coffee can be traced back directly to the Revolutionary War. Fashionable teas had remained the beverage of choice for cultured Americans until the Boston Tea Party in 1773, when colonists angered by high British taxes dumped chests of tea into Boston Harbor, an act of defiance that ignited the War of Independence—and caused most Americans to prove their patriotism by switching from tea to coffee. As John Adams wrote to Abigail about stopping for refreshment after a long ride and being told by the proprietor, " '(W)e have renounced all Tea in this place. I can't make tea, but I'le make you Coffee.' Accordingly I have drank Coffee every afternoon since, and have borne it very well."

The effects of coffee have been debated for hundreds of

years. In 1674, for example, English women complained that this "nauseous Puddle-water . . . has Eunucht our Husbands. . . . [T]hey are become as impotent as Age." While at almost precisely the same moment a tract written by an otherwise unknown M.P. celebrated its virtues, "'Tis extolled for drying up the Crudities of the Stomack, and for expelling Fumes out of the Head. Excellent Berry! Which can cleanse the English-man's Stomak of Flegm, and expel Giddinesse out of his Head."

For much of recent history it was generally accepted that while coffee certainly had a pleasing taste and was very useful in keeping people awake and alert, it could cause some serious problems and really should be used in moderation. In fact, no one knew with scientific certainty exactly what health problems or benefits, if any, were the consequence of drinking coffee. But that began changing in the 1960s.

While most medical studies begin with a specific premise to be tested, a hypothesis, a tremendous amount of information can be gleaned from statistical analysis of information collected with no specific point of view. It's an examination of real-world behaviors and results and is known as epidemiological research. One of the largest of these observational studies was conducted by the Kaiser-Permanente Medical Care Program. KP had been founded during World War II as a prepayment medical plan for employees of Kaiser Shipyards and had expanded coverage after the war. In many ways it was the model for the HMOs that would follow. During the 1960s KP began a study to determine which medical tests had value and which did not. This involved setting up a computerized database to store and analyze information gathered from decades of health checkup examinations. Although the computers were rudimentary, the database made it possible to glean a tremendous amount of statistical evidence concerning a variety of conditions.

One of those initial studies was essentially a search for new heart attack predictors. According to Dr. Gary D. Friedman, who believed that by analyzing that mountain of information researchers could determine which behaviors increased the risk that a person would have a heart attack, "Counting all historic queries and measurements we had compiled data on about five hundred different items and some of them would prove predictive of heart attacks. For example, we found that abstinence from alcohol predicted a *higher* risk for heart attacks to that seen in light or moderate drinkers. This was not a pre-study hypothesis and it led us to further explore alcohol and health."

Another study from that same database, first published in 1992 and updated in 2006, reported an inverse relationship between drinking coffee and liver cirrhosis. This was not totally unexpected, but the extent of the impact was somewhat surprising. Coffee lowered the level of liver enzymes in the blood; astonishingly, the study found that the more coffee individuals drank, the less chance they had of developing alcoholic cirrhosis. Each daily cup accounted for a 20 percent reduction in risk. For example, people who drink a lot of alcohol could reduce their chance of developing cirrhosis 40 percent by drinking two cups of regular coffee a day and by an astounding 80 percent by drinking four cups of regular coffee a day. But I caution my friends and the lay public that this is not a license to drink an excessive amount of alcohol and then protect your liver by drinking regular coffee. It will likely protect the liver, but that amount of alcohol can damage the brain, lead to heart failure, pancreatitis, and impotence, and of course it can ruin someone's professional career and lead to untold family turmoil.

This was a startling discovery; the evidence was strong that coffee could reduce chances of alcoholic cirrhosis, but the analysis couldn't determine why it was true. "Epidemiology doesn't determine mechanisms," explains Dr. Arthur Klatsky, a cardiologist and investigator in the Kaiser Permanente Research Division who conducted the study. "It usually shows only associations. Like most other people, I was surprised at the strength of the apparent protection. When you see something that is reduced 60 percent, 70 percent, 80 percent that is a very major reduction risk. And that's what we found in the relationship between heavy coffee drinking and the likelihood of developing cirrhosis. But it's very important to emphasize that the best way to reduce the risk of alcoholic cirrhosis is to limit the alcohol intake, not to cover heavy alcoholic consumption by drinking coffee."

As Dr. Klatsky points out, the numbers tell a story, but they do so without any details. The data doesn't report which type of coffee people drink, whether they add anything to it, whether it's filtered, or even if it's caffeinated or decaffeinated. All that is known is the number of cups of coffee people drink every day and how that impacts disease. Personally, Dr. Klatsky reports that he has "two cups of coffee in the morning and sometimes a cup at noon. Three is my maximum. Otherwise it keeps me awake."

Dr. Klatsky's research helped stir the growing interest in the health benefits of coffee. While coffee has been prized for its value as a stimulant for centuries, few people suspected it might have additional benefits. And since coffee, unlike most drugs, can't be patented—not even by Starbucks—there had been little financial incentive for private industry to support the enormous costs of research. So most studies about the effects of coffee have been conducted by large institutions and public health agencies and paid for by the government.

Perhaps because of Klatsky's unexpected findings about liver cirrhosis, many of the larger studies have investigated the effects of coffee on the liver. In August 2007, for example, the preeminent journal *Hepatology* reported that ten different studies conducted in Europe and Asia demonstrated that men and women who regularly drink coffee have a significantly reduced chance of developing liver cancer. Liver cancer is an especially virulent disease, with almost thirty-five thousand Americans diagnosed each year. Worldwide, primary liver cancer (cancer arising from within the liver) is the third leading cause of cancer mortality. One million individuals succumb to it each year. As it turns out, drinking coffee apparently greatly reduces the odds of being one of those people. The studies included approximately 240,000 people, among them 2,260 diagnosed with the disease, and showed that people who drink at least several cups of coffee daily had less than half the chance of being diagnosed with liver cancer than study participants who drink no coffee. In fact, the odds drop by 23 percent with each daily cup.

An Italian meta-analysis of sixteen high-quality studies published in *Clinical Gastroenterology and Hepatology* in 2013 reported that coffee consumption reduced risk of hepatocellular carcinoma, the most common type of liver cancer, by about 40 percent, adding that some data indicated that drinking three or more cups daily reduced that risk by more than 50 percent.

As in Dr. Klatsky's cirrhosis study there was no attempt made to determine the reason for this protection, although there is some speculation that coffee affects liver enzymes.

Why or how it works remains somewhat of a mystery. What we have learned is that coffee drinkers have lower levels of liver enzymes in the blood, less liver fibrosis (scarring), a dramatic reduction in the rate of hospitalization from chronic liver disease, and, as mentioned above, a substantially lower risk of developing primary liver cancer.

Another study conducted by investigators at the Harvard School of Public Health and Beth Israel Deaconess Medical Center showed that coffee drinkers have high levels of plasma adiponectin. Low levels of plasma adiponectin have been shown to be linked with aggressive liver disease. Coffee drinkers also have low levels of C-reactive protein (CRP), increased levels of which signal a greater risk for developing atherosclerotic heart disease, which often manifests as a heart attack. Coffee's effect on glucose metabolism may be what makes it responsible for other vitally important benefits.

While previous studies had failed to find a link between drinking coffee and prostate cancer, a 2009 study funded by the National Institutes of Health closely followed fifty thousand male health professionals for two decades and found that men who drank six or more cups of either caffeinated or decaffeinated coffee daily reduced their chances of developing advanced prostate cancer by an astounding 60 percent; in addition, men who enjoyed four or five cups saw a 25 percent reduction, and drinking three cups lowered risk by 20 percent, compared with people who did not drink coffee. Harvard's Kathryn Wilson, one of the authors of the study, speculating on why this might be true, suggested, "Coffee has effects on insulin and glucose metabolism as well as [on] sex hormone levels, all of which play a role in prostate cancer."

If all coffee did was reduce the risk of a variety of liver diseases it would still be very valuable, but the very promising news is that there is a rapidly growing body of evidence that it has many other real benefits. Perhaps most exciting is its potential to impact type 2 or adult-onset diabetes. Coffee, by virtue of being insulin sensitizing, meaning it improves the body's response to insulin, decreases the risk of developing type 2 diabetes by 40 percent—if one drinks six cups of it (but it can be regular or decaf).

We are facing a worldwide epidemic of this very dangerous disease. It is estimated that almost 250 million people worldwide suffer from diabetes and that the vast majority of them have been diagnosed with type 2, which can lead to an array of serious problems. Researchers at the Harvard School of Public Health and Brigham and Women's Hospital conducted an eighteen-year study beginning in 1980 in which they tracked 125,000 people. The results, published in *Annals of Internal Medicine* in 2004, were impressive: People who drink coffee regularly can significantly reduce their risk of type 2 diabetes. Men who drank six or more cups daily reduced their chances of being diagnosed with adult-onset diabetes by 54 percent; women who drank the same amount reduced their risk by about 30 percent. As lead researcher Dr. Frank Hu explained, "We don't know exactly why coffee is beneficial for diabetes. . . . Coffee contains large amounts of antioxidants such as chlorogenic acid and tocopherols, and minerals such as magnesium. All of these components have been shown to improve insulin sensitivity and affect glucose metabolism."

Those findings were confirmed by a meta-analysis conducted at Australia's University of Sydney. A team of international researchers examined eighteen studies involving more than 450,000 participants and reported in *Archives of Internal Medicine* in 2009, "Every additional cup of coffee consumed in a day was associated with a 7 percent reduction in the excess risk of diabetes."

In the world of coffee, quality is in the cup of the beholder, but for researchers it's simply a matter of quantity. Both of these studies demonstrated that quantity makes a difference. The philosopher Voltaire was purported to enjoy as many as fifty to seventy-two small cups of coffee daily—and died in 1778 at the age of eighty-three. While that certainly seems to be a bit extreme, participants in the Harvard study who drank six or more cups daily saw by far the greatest reduction in risk, an extraordinary 50 percent, while adults who had four or five cups reduced their chances of getting diabetes by 30 percent and people who consumed fewer than four normal-sized cups daily reduced their risk by 2–7 percent. Interestingly, that Harvard study also showed that women gained no additional protection by drinking five or more cups a day.

Both the Harvard and Australian studies found different—but still valuable—outcomes when coffee drinkers chose decaf: Drinking four or more cups of decaffeinated coffee daily reduced the risk of developing diabetes by a still impressive 25 percent for men and by 15 percent for women. Clearly there are benefits no matter what type of coffee you drink—so long as you drink a fair amount of it.

Further confirming this link was an eleven-year study

beginning in 1986 conducted at the University of Minnesota examining the relationship between drinking coffee and diabetes in postmenopausal women. Since type 2 diabetes most often occurs in people older than forty-five, postmeno-pausal women are an especially affected group. This study reported that women who drank six or more cups of any type of coffee reduced their chances of being diagnosed with diabetes by 22 percent. There are a lot of people who see that number—six cups!—and complain that if they drank that much coffee they'd be awake for the following two months, but an especially puzzling aspect of that study showed that women who drank six or more cups of decaffeinated coffee actually saw a greater reduction, 33 percent, in risk.

There are a lot of different theories as to why men and women consistently have been shown to have different responses to coffee; the present theory is that a woman's hormones—or, more often, hormone-replacement drugs in postmenopausal women—mitigate the effect.

Another common belief is that because coffee is a stimulant, meaning it speeds up the heart, people with heart conditions should be advised to carefully limit the amount of coffee they drink. Actually, the evidence is somewhat mixed. A 2008 Nurses' Health Study published in the *Annals of Internal Medicine* followed more than forty thousand male health professionals for eighteen years and reported that men who drank five or more cups of coffee a day reduced their risk of dying from heart disease by 44 percent.

According to a Beth Israel Deaconess Medical Center study published in the *American Heart Journal* in 2009, that reduction in risk is seen even in people who have already suffered heart attacks. The Stockholm Heart Epidemiology Program enrolled more than thirteen hundred men and women who had a confirmed heart attack between 1992 and 1994. Eight years later those patients who normally drank four to five cups of coffee daily had reduced their risk of suffering a fatal heart attack almost by half over those people who averaged less than a cup a day, while those men and women who enjoyed one to three cups of coffee daily reduced that risk by about a third.

A Harvard study conducted in collaboration with researchers from the Universidad Autónoma de Madrid investigated the possible link between coffee and strokes in women. Using data from a twenty-four-year-long Nurses' Health Study, in which eighty-three thousand women regularly completed questionnaires about their eating habits, including coffee consumption, researchers discovered that women who drank two or more cups a day reduced the risk of stroke by 19 percent—and the more coffee they drank the greater the reduction in risk. Women who did not smoke reported even more impressive benefits: Nonsmoking women who enjoyed four or more cups of coffee a day reduced the incidence of stroke by 43 percent! This level of risk reduction is equal to the impact of some of the best-selling drugs in the world.

As has been demonstrated in other studies, it is not simply the caffeine that contributes to this result. In fact, people who chose to drink caffeinated tea or soft drinks did not enjoy the same benefits, while women who drank two or more cups of decaffeinated coffee did show a reduced risk for stroke. According to epidemiologist Esther Lopez-Garcia, one of the directors of the Harvard study, "This finding supports the hypothesis that components in coffee other than caffeine may be responsible for the potential benefit of coffee on stroke risk."

Coffee drinkers
have a substantially
lowered risk of heart attacks
and do not have an increased
risk of cardiac arrhythmias.

Another Kaiser Permanente study investigated the long-held belief that people with cardiac arrhythmias, a rapid or irregular heartbeat, should avoid or at least substantially limit the amount of coffee they drink. The thinking is logical: Coffee is a stimulant that speeds up the heart, so people whose heart can go out of rhythm should avoid it. But in this one study, at least, the result was quite different. Dr. Klatsky and his colleagues analyzed data collected from more than 130,000 participants over a seven-year period and found that people who drank at least four cups of coffee daily reduced their risk of being admitted to a hospital for a heart rhythm disturbance by almost 20 percent. This study, presented at the American Heart Association's fiftieth Annual Conference on Cardiovascular Disease Epidemiology and Prevention in 2010, found that the reduced risk extended to the various types of rhythm disturbance. Dr. Klatsky admitted that the results of this study were surprising: "The conventional wisdom is that coffee can cause palpitations and it can cause rhythm problems. I think, though, that conventional wisdom is not always right and the data that were available before this study do not support the idea that moderate amounts of coffee provoke rhythm problems."

Dr. Klatsky added, "we're not going to recommend that people drink coffee to prevent rhythm problems," but that people who drink a moderate amount of coffee "can be reassured that they are not increasing their risk of significant heart rhythm problems."

Regular coffee drinking also appears to reduce one's chances of getting colon and other cancers. The 2010 NIH-AARP Diet and Health Study published in the *American Journal for Clinical Nutrition*, which followed almost half a million men and women for more than ten years, found that those people who drank more than four cups of coffee daily reduced their risk of colon cancer by about 16 percent. That same study also found that people who drank tea did not see similar benefits.

In 2014, a smaller study conducted by researchers from the University of Southern California's Norris Comprehensive Cancer Center tracked the coffee consumption of 8,500 Israelis, the majority of whom had been diagnosed with colon cancer, and reported that compared with people who did not drink coffee, people who drank one or two cups daily reduced their risk by 22 percent while those who drank three or more cups lowered their risk by 59 percent. There is no scientific explanation for this. The results confirmed those from a 2007 Japanese study published in the *International Journal of Cancer* that found that women who drank three or more cups of coffee every day saw their risk of being diagnosed with colon cancer reduced by about half.

Additional studies have found that coffee may even cut chances of being diagnosed with other types of cancer. For example, researchers at Harvard Medical School and Brigham and Women's Hospital analyzed data collected from 110,000 people over more than two decades and found that women who drank more than three cups of caffeinated coffee daily had a 20 percent lower risk of developing basal cell carcinoma, the most common form of skin cancer, compared with women who did not drink coffee. Men saw their risk reduced by 9 percent, but there was no association with other and more potentially lethal forms of skin cancer. Another Japanese study, this one following 38,000 people and published by *Epidemiology*, concluded that people who drank at least one cup of coffee a day saw their risk of getting cancers of the mouth, pharynx, and esophagus reduced by more than half.

While once again the mechanisms aren't yet known, there is no doubt that drinking coffee regularly reduces the risk of being diagnosed with several common cancers, including primary liver cancer, colon cancer, skin cancer, endometrial cancer, and metastatic prostatecancer. There is no magic formula (this many cups has this effect on this cancer), but the impact is real and significant.

What if I told you that drinking might make you smarter? Some people, I suspect, would respond by suggesting I'd better drink more coffee. But the evidence does appear to indicate that coffee may be very good for your mental health. As Honoré de Balzac wrote almost two centuries ago, "As soon as coffee is in your stomach, there is a general commotion. Ideas begin to move . . . similes arise, the paper is covered. Coffee is your ally and writing ceases to be a struggle." Numerous controlled trials have shown that coffee does seem to have a positive affect on cognitive function. It appears to be able to stimulate mood and various brain functions by blocking an inhibitory neurotransmitter in the brain. It has been shown to specifically reduce chances of being diagnosed with Parkinson's disease and dementia, specifically Alzheimer's.

A study published in 2000 in the *Journal of the American Medical Association* analyzed three decades of data from 8,004 participants in the Honolulu Heart Program and reported that people who did not drink coffee had five times more risk of eventually being diagnosed with Parkinson's than people who consumed three or more cups of coffee a day. A 2010 meta-analysis of twenty-six studies conducted by the Center for Evidence-Based Medicine at the University of Lisbon "confirmed an inverse association between caffeine intake and the risk of Parkinson's Disease." These twenty-six studies concluded that regularly drinking three or more cups of coffee reduces chances of getting this neurological disease by 25 percent, and drinking more coffee further reduces that risk. And a 2007 Duke University Medical Center study of the relation of smoking, drinking coffee, and the disease stated flatly, "Individuals with Parkinson's Disease were also less likely to drink large amounts of coffee." Numerous other studies have shown that the more coffee you drink, the less likely it is you will be diagnosed with Parkinson's. This is true for both men and women, although a two-decade-long study of 77,000 women found that those women not taking post-menopausal hormones saw the same reduction in risk as men, but women taking estrogens lost some of that protection if they drank a large amount of coffee.

While the evidence linking coffee to a reduced risk of Alzheimer's isn't as clear-cut as its effect against other ailments, there have been several good studies in which it appears to have a positive impact in preventing the onset or progression of the disease. A Scandinavian study published in 2009 in the *Journal of Alzheimer's* analyzed data collected from about 1,400 people for two decades and reported that those participants who consumed three to five cups of coffee daily reduced their risk of being diagnosed with dementia or Alzheimer's by 65 percent. While other studies showed somewhat less dramatic results, they have consistently indicated that caffeinated coffee prevents memory decline in older people and reduces the risk of developing full-blown Alzheimer's.

Intrigued by these findings, German and French researchers reported in 2014 that regular doses of caffeine helped prevent the buildup of tau protein deposits in laboratory mice. These deposits, which clog up the insides of brain cells, are a hallmark of Alzheimer's. This study mirrored results from a 2011 University of South Florida study, as reported in *Medical News Today,* that found that coffee "wards off Alzheimer's" because it stimulates an unknown factor in a critical protein to put off development of the disease.

All the various ways in which coffee affects the brain really aren't known; we just know that it does. It has been shown that coffee stimulates the release of dopamine, a neurotransmitter known to produce feelings of well-being. In fact, there are many researchers who believe that its ability to produce dopamine accounts for coffee's worldwide popularity. But it does seem to have other direct ramifications: Coffee appears to offer at least some protection against clinical depression and suicide. An NIH-supported study conducted by the Department of Nutrition at the Harvard School of Public Health published in 2011 analyzed data from about 50,000 women who were free of depression when they began participating and were followed for as long as twenty-five years. "In 3 cohort studies, 2 from the United States and 1 from Finland," investigators reported, "strong inverse associations have been reported between coffee consumption and suicide, which is strongly associated with depression." This study found that women who drank four or more cups of coffee a day reduced their risk of depression by 20 percent—intriguingly, women who drank decaffeinated coffee or other beverages with caffeine showed almost no benefit. Data collected from 86,000 nurses from 1980 to 1990 and published in 1996 by the *Journal of the American Medical Association* seemed to confirm this finding by showing that women who drank four or more

Those who drink coffee
have a lower chance of developing
both Alzheimer's dementia
and Parkinson's disease.

cups of a coffee a day reduced their risk of committing suicide by more than half.

Not only does coffee seem to prevent or slow the loss of certain brain functions, it also may make you smarter, thinner, and improve your physical performance. As much as that sounds like a product that might have been sold from the back of a covered wagon by a snake oil salesman, there is real scientific research to support those claims. A 2008 report from the British Nutrition Foundation reviewed sixteen studies on healthy, well-rested subjects and found, "14 reported benefits relating to caffeine consumption, including improved alertness, short-term recall and reaction time. There were also consistent findings for positive mood. . . ." It is known that coffee causes chemical reactions in the brain that enable neurons to increase function. One result of that, as the *New York Times* reported in 2014, is that coffee can help increase test scores. It might not actually be making people smarter, but just be improving their power of recall and the speed at which their brain functions.

Any product that makes you thinner is bound to attract a lot of attention. Coffee can be a mixed bean where that is concerned. Caffeine is among the few natural substances known to burn fat, and small studies have reported that it can increase the rate at which the body burns fat by as much as 10 percent in obese people and 29 percent in thin individuals. It's for that reason that just about every fat-burning supplement on the market contains a substantial amount of caffeine. Of course, it is important to emphasize that many people load up their coffee with all types of high caloric additions, and a large coffee with whipped cream, sugar, flavored syrups, and other substances can easily weigh in at more than five hundred calories—far more than it will burn. So while no one would consider coffee a weight-loss substance, black coffee or even coffee with a little milk or sweetener added can fit nicely into a healthy diet.

There is considerably more evidence that coffee helps improve physical performance. Until recently, for example, the Olympic Games Committee included coffee among its controlled substances, which meant athletes could drink only a small, designated amount. As *Fitness Magazine* reported in 2005, "Caffeine acts as a central nervous system stimulant, producing effects—such as increased heart rate and blood pressure—that can make you feel more alert and energetic. Caffeine can also function as an ergogenic aid, meaning that its physiological effects enhance athletic performance. Most experts agree that caffeine's impact on the nervous system alters one's perceived level of exertion, making your workout seem easier and allowing you to exercise longer before feeling tired." A 2004 meta-analysis published in the *Journal of Sports Nutrition* that included forty double-blind studies found that caffeinated coffee increased performance on exercise tests by about 12 percent. According to Dr. Terry Graham, of Canada's University of Guelph and a longtime researcher of the value of coffee to athletes, "What caffeine likely does is stimulate the brain and nervous system to do things differently. That may include signaling you to ignore fatigue or recruit extra units of muscle for intense athletic performance. Caffeine may even have a direct effect on muscles themselves, causing them to produce a stronger contraction."

Also writing in the *Journal of Sports Nutrition,* researcher M. Doherty reported that a 180-pound male, after drinking five cups of coffee, "significantly increased muscle endurance during [a] brief, intense workout" and that for a 130-pound woman who is a recreational runner "three cups of coffee resulted in significantly greater anaerobic metabolism and improved athletic performance."

While the mechanism isn't known precisely, the benefits to physical performance certainly are. One major league baseball clubhouse manager reported that during a game some players will drink as many as six cups of coffee to maintain total focus and enhance success.

This increased focus and attention may help explain another apparent benefit of coffee that is especially surprising: Coffee seems to reduce the risk that an individual will die from injuries and accidents. In 2012, the *New England Journal of Medicine* published a study in which researchers analyzed data collected from about 400,000 people for more than a decade in the NIH-AARP Diet and Health Study and concluded, "this large prospective cohort study showed significant inverse associations of coffee consumption with death from all causes and specifically with deaths from . . . injuries and accidents." This result was consistent with similar findings in several other large studies. In some cases the value of caffeinated coffee is pretty obvious: A 2013 Australian study published in the *British Medical Journal* tracked about one thousand long-haul truck drivers, approximately half of whom recently had been in an accident. It is well-known that fatigue is a primary cause of automobile and truck accidents. Drivers who used some form of caffeine—which included tea and energy drinks—reduced the chances of being in an accident by 63 percent. In fact, this association is so compelling that some automotive manufacturers actually have added a steaming cup of coffee icon to their dashboard warning lights;

Mercedes Attention Assist system creates a driver profile that enables sensors to measure driver alertness. After a certain deviation the coffee cup icon appears, suggesting drivers are not focused and should pull over for a cup of caffeinated coffee.

Recent research also seems to indicate that coffee may help prevent gum disease and even cavities. Let me repeat that because most often the only thing people know about coffee is that it may stain teeth: Coffee may be good for your teeth. In a 2014 study published in the *Journal of Periodontology*, researchers at the Boston University Henry M. Goldman School of Dental Medicine examined the health data collected from 1,152 men over a thirty-year period as part of the Department of Veterans Affairs Dental Longitudinal Study and found that "[h]igher coffee consumption was associated with a small but significant reduction in the number of teeth with periodontal bone loss." There also is some evidence that coffee will prevent tooth decay by fighting mouth bacteria. The *Journal of Agricultural and Food Chemistry* reported that the antibacterial properties of several chemical compounds found in coffee, especially trigonelline, stop bacteria from attacking tooth enamel. A 2009 Indian study of one thousand random participants who were followed for more than three decades—funded by several coffee associations—concluded that people who drink black coffee can significantly reduce the incidence of dental cavities, but additives including milk and sugar eliminate most of that protection.

And while there have been few human studies, the journal *Molecular Vision* reported in 2010 that in animal studies scientists at the University of Maryland had found that caffeine could prevent the formation of cataracts. A similar experiment conducted in Sweden in 2013, in which caffeine eye drops were used, produced the same level of encouraging results.

Perhaps not surprising is the fact that coffee appears to reduce significantly the formation of gallstones. Gallstones are small, pebble-like, hard particles that form in the gallbladder. They can obstruct a duct coming out of the gallbladder, called the cystic duct, and lead to inflammation of the gallbladder, a condition called acute cholecystitis. On occasion, the gallstones can migrate down the common bile duct and get stuck, where the pancreatic duct and the common bile duct enter the small bowel. This complication is called acute pancreatitis and has up to a 10 percent mortality rate. The Health Professionals Follow-up Study published in 1999 analyzed data collected over a decade from 46,008 men without a history of gallstone disease and reported that men who drank between two and four cups of caffeinated coffee a day reduced the incidence of gallstones by 45 percent, while those people who drank decaffeinated coffee did not see a similar result.

A companion study published three years later analyzed data from the Nurses' Health Study—in which almost ninety thousand women participated for almost three decades—and reported that women who drank two to three cups of caffeinated coffee a day had a 22 percent lower risk of developing gallstones, and drinking even more coffee only slightly increased that protection.

There is no longer any doubt that coffee offers significant health benefits, but in many areas the reasons for that simply haven't been found or proved. Coffee consists of hundreds of component chemicals, among them potassium, magnesium, and vitamin E, and is rich in antioxidants, especially chlorogenic acid. Coffee also contains kahweol and cafestol. These constituents have been shown to abrogate experimental, induced liver injury in laboratory animals. In fact, most people living in our part of the world get more antioxidants from coffee than from all of the fruits and vegetables they eat combined. The coffee bean is known to contain more than one thousand compounds that might have some effect on mortality. In mysterious ways these and other constituents of coffee combine to offer this varied protection. As researchers at the University of Sydney reported after concluding that coffee reduced the risk of diabetes, "Our findings suggest that any protective effects of coffee . . . are unlikely to be solely the effects of caffeine, but rather, as has been speculated previously, they likely involve a broader range of chemical constituents present in these beverages, such as magnesium, lignans and chlorogenic acids."

The primary component, of course, is caffeine. Caffeine is a chemical stimulant actually found in more than sixty different plants. Chemists lovingly refer to it as trimethylxanthine. It acts mostly on the brain and the nervous system, creating a temporary boost of energy and focus. Certainly the presence of caffeine may contribute to some of the many health benefits. Indeed there is about three-and-a-half times as much caffeine in an eight-ounce cup of coffee as there is in the same sized serving of tea or cola or in an ounce of chocolate. But it is worth noting that tea and colas that contain caffeine have not been shown to have all the remarkable health benefits of coffee. While it is not generally known, there is as much or more caffeine in a single dose of common pain relievers like Anacin or Excedrin as there is in a large cup of coffee.

One of the properties of caffeine is that it gives a boost to other important chemicals. When you drink it, it is rapidly absorbed into the bloodstream and goes to work. Some researchers believe it is caffeine's ability to constrict blood vessels, thus reducing blood flow, that contributes to its effects. By blocking a neurotransmitter named adensoine, caffeine magnifies the effect of other neurotransmitters. For example, it has been shown to increase levels of dopamine, the neurotransmitter that helps control the brain's centers of rewards and pleasure. It injects adrenalin into your system to provide an energy boost. It appears to help regulate the levels of liver enzymes in the blood. And, as mentioned, it magnifies the effectiveness of common painkillers like aspirin and acetaminophen and helps bring rapid relief from headaches and, in some situations, asthma.

But as with absolutely everything else produced by mother nature, there are some effects of coffee that can cause problems. As the 1674 Women's Petition Against Coffee warned, "Coffee leads men to trifle away their time, scald their chops and spend their money, all for a little base, black, thick, nasty, bitter, stinking nauseous puddle water." And while it's not quite that bad, coffee has been blamed for a wide variety of ailments, including stunting growth, a variety of heart problems, and even cancer. But most of those claims have been disproved.

However, there are potential health issues associated with coffee, especially with drinking more than two or cups a day. The first, of course, is that it can be addictive, meaning that once you start drinking coffee and your system gets used to it, it's very difficult to stop drinking it—and if you do, sometimes even for a day, the physical repercussions of withdrawal can include headaches and nausea. It can make you feel unusually tired and even depressed. Those people who drink more coffee than their system can easily tolerate may become overstimulated; too much caffeine can cause nervousness, a rapid heartbeat, excitability, insomnia, and worsening heartburn. Interestingly, heartburn can also be seen with decaffeinated coffee. The reason for heartburn is that the peptides present in the roasted beans from which coffee is brewed lead to increased acid secretion by specialized cells in the stomach.

It is the effect of coffee, and for that matter any beverage containing caffeine, on the heart that has made people wary. Caffeinated coffee makes the heart beat faster, that's a fact. But what hasn't been demonstrated is that a rapid heartbeat will cause health issues. According to Dr. Murray Mittleman, director of the Cardiovascular Epidemiology Research Unit at Beth Israel Deaconess Medical Center, animal studies have shown that caffeinated coffee can acutely raise blood pressure, and, "[s]ince high blood pressure is a risk factor for many types of cardiovascular disease, researchers assumed that coffee would be harmful. But several studies have shown that although there is an increase in blood pressure shortly after consumption there are health benefits over the long-term. Coffee contains many active compounds, including antioxidants, that may explain how coffee lowers the risk of Type 2 diabetes, and in turn may lower the risk of developing heart failure." Dr. Mittleman and his colleagues analyzed data from five large studies that included 140,000 men and women, most of them in Scandinavia, and reported that low levels of coffee consumption essentially had little effect on the risk of heart failure while four or five cups a day could be associated with an increased risk.

The American Heart Association points out that while there is conflicting data about the effects of drinking four or more cups a day, there is no evidence that drinking two cups causes any problem and, in fact, doing so might be beneficial for your heart.

Similar results were seen in several other good studies. In the Women's Health Study 33,638 women older than forty-five were followed for sixteen years, and the data showed that drinking coffee could not be associated with an increased risk of atrial fibrillation.

One of the biggest concerns about coffee is that it contributes to the loss of calcium and bone density, leading to osteoporosis, especially in women. Caffeine is known to make it more difficult for your body to absorb calcium, and calcium builds strong bones. The evidence about this is mixed. In 2002 the journal *Food and Chemical Toxicology* reported that caffeine consumption did result in a small decrease in calcium absorption, but that minor decrease might easily be offset by adding one or two tablespoons of milk.

A Swedish study of seven hundred elderly men and women published in *Nutrition and Metabolism* in 2010 showed that drinking about four cups of coffee a day was associated with a small decrease in bone density in men but not in women and concluded, "This study further states that, similar to other studies, there is consistently no link between caffeine consumption and a decrease in bone mineral density in women."

Other studies have shown that for a small number of women drinking more than four cups of caffeinated coffee a day may exacerbate the progression of osteoporosis. The National Osteoporosis Foundation recommends that women keep coffee consumption at a moderate level.

There also have been some concerns about the effect of coffee, specifically caffeine, on pregnant women, the great fear being that it affects the fetus. The American College of Obstetricians and Gynecologists currently advises that a cup of coffee a day will not increase the risk of miscarriage or premature birth. According to Dr. William Barth, chairman of the ACOG's Committee on Obstetric Practice, "After a review of the scientific evidence to date, daily moderate caffeine consumption doesn't appear to have any major impact in causing miscarriage or preterm birth."

But clearly the almost universal effect of caffeinated coffee is that, like any stimulant, it keeps people awake. That can be a very good thing when you're driving or have work to complete, but insomnia or sleep deprivation can result in some serious problems. Regular sleep is essential for good health. In addition to simply making you feel good, it provides an opportunity for various systems in your body to function optimally. According to Dr. Shelby Freedman Harris, director of behavioral sleep medicine at New York's Montefiore Hospital Sleep-Wake Disorder Centers, "When you're sleeping you're regulating hormone levels, you're regulating insulin levels, your blood pressure is being kept under control, there are a lot of things going on, and if you're not getting enough sleep you're throwing these things out of whack."

The half-life of caffeine in the body is approximately six hours, meaning its effect is diminished by half in that period of time. That's why many people can have their last cup of coffee for the day in the early afternoon and sleep quite well that night. For some people, though, even a small amount of caffeine in their system can prevent them from gaining the benefits of deep sleep.

And finally it was Balzac who pointed out another purported troubling aspect of coffee: "Coffee is a great power in my life; I have observed its effects on an epic scale. Coffee roasts your insides. Many people claim coffee inspires them, but as everybody knows, coffee only makes boring people more boring! Think about it. Although more grocery stores in Paris are staying open until midnight, few writers are actually becoming more spiritual."

While the overall health benefits of coffee have now be proven without any doubt, the question still remains how much coffee you should be drinking. The obvious answer is no more than your system can tolerate; if it keeps you up all night or makes you nervous or anxious, you're drinking too much. If you're adding hundreds of calories with creams and syrups it's probably too much. I know a man who recently celebrated his ninetieth birthday and for many years he drank an amazing forty cups of coffee and smoked two packs of cigarettes a day; as he says, "My feet went months without touching the ground." Since then he has reduced his coffee and given up cigarettes completely and still goes to work everyday. Another person I know can hardly tolerate the one cup of coffee he drinks each day when we meet at our local coffee shop, although perhaps as Balzac surmised the coffee is good but it is the company he doesn't tolerate well!

One reason it's difficult to make any kind of recommendation about how much coffee it is healthy to drink in one day is the fact that not all coffee beans are created equally, and there are almost as many different ways to prepare it as there are different types. While various teas and wines have different names, usually based on their origin, taste, and effect, among most people coffee is known simply as coffee. In fact, there are two broad classifications of coffee: arabica and robusta. Arabica is mild and aromatic and accounts for about 70 percent of the world's coffee production. Robusta is a heartier bean with a much higher caffeine content and is used primarily in blends and instant coffee. There are about seventy coffee-exporting countries, and the taste of each coffee bean is different, sometimes just a bit or as much as a great deal, depending on the soil, the amount of rainfall, and other natural variables. Kenyan coffee, for example, has a full-bodied rich fragrance with a sharp, fruity acidity, while Colombian supremo is known for its delicate, aromatic sweetness. Brazil is the world's leading coffee exporter, followed by Vietnam, Indonesia, Colombia, and Ethiopia. In each of these countries coffee contributes significantly to the nation's economy and financial stability. Incidentally, the world's most expensive coffee isn't found at your local coffee shop: it's called Black Ivory coffee and comes primarily from Thailand. Well, actually it comes through elephants. Elephants eat arabica beans but they don't digest them; instead these beans take several days to pass through the elephants' digestive system, during which time they are fermenting. They are finally excreted and collected and sold at five-star hotels for about $70 a cup. Kopi luwak, or civet coffee, comes from the excretions of a civet, a small mammal found mostly in Indonesia. Because it is so expensive, starting at about $160 a pound, producers were breeding civets and keeping them caged, although there has been a movement to prevent that from happening. But I think it is quite accurate to report that with rare exceptions your daily coffee hasn't been in any other stomachs!

The way coffee is processed and even how it is brewed will make a difference in its taste, but also may make a difference in its effect. The paper filters used to brew coffee will absorb almost all of a substance called cafestol, which is a potent stimulator of LDL cholesterol levels, while coffee made with a French press or simply boiled will contain all of the original cafestol. Each of the series of steps from picking the cherry to its being poured into your cup can affect your coffee—although because most studies are epidemiological they do not differentiate between the numerous types nor the way it has been prepared.

Recommendations about how much coffee to drink vary. Personally, I love coffee and will drink as many as four or five cups a day, usually with skim milk or black but without a sweetener. According to Dr. van Dam of the Harvard School of Public Health, as long as your body can tolerate it there are no negative effects associated with drinking up to six eight-ounce cups of caffeinated coffee (one hundred milligrams) a day. The Mayo Clinic reports that four cups "appears to be safe for most healthy adults." The American Medical Association points out that two to three eight-ounce cups is about average but that ten cups is an excessive amount. The AMA also reminds Americans that when coffee is loaded with sweeteners and taste enhancers it can silently add to obesity. The U.S. Food and Drug Administration reports that four hundred milligrams of caffeine, found in four cups of coffee, is a safe amount of caffeine for healthy adults—then reminds people that they might also be getting caffeine from a variety of other products, including soda, chocolate, and even some gum.

So the best answer is that there is no best answer. For most Americans the amount of coffee you are drinking now is the right amount. If it doesn't cause you any physical distress please enjoy your coffee. As the diplomat Prince Tallyrand wrote, "Suave molecules of Mocha stir up your blood, without causing excess heat; the organ of thought receives from it a feeling of sympathy; work becomes easier and you will sit down without distress to your principle repast which will restore your body and afford you a calm, delicious night."

Fortunately for me I happen to love the aroma and flavor of coffee. For years, I have stopped on the way to work at 6:00 A.M. at a favorite java shop. I usually get a tall, dark, rich, robust coffee and sit down with three friends for ten to fifteen minutes before getting back into the car. By 5:00 P.M., I've had another two or three cups of this magical elixir.

2

THE MYSTERIOUS
CASE OF VITAMIN D

I f the legendary detective Sherlock Holmes was instead a
scientist, undoubtedly he would have been fascinated by . . .
The Strange Case of Vitamin D! Vitamin D is an imposter; it
is disguised as a vitamin. Not only that, its value is cloaked in
mystery: While we know what it does, we have little evidence
of its actual effect. There really is only one thing about this
substance that we know for certain: Everybody needs it, and
many people need a lot more than they're getting in their diet.

At one point I was with three colleagues from Harvard
Medical School on a long flight to Singapore, where we were
to teach a postgraduate medical course. These three distin-
guished professors represented the specialties of cardiology,
oncology, and nephrology. During our conversation I asked
them if they were taking any vitamins. Two of them told me
that the only vitamin they took was vitamin D3. The third
doctor, the cardiologist, said that he didn't take any vitamin
D, but he felt quite healthy and therefore didn't feel he needed
it. I responded to him that I took 2,000—4,000 IU (international units) a day and implored him to see his primary care

physician and have his vitamin D3 level checked as soon as we got back to Boston.

A few days after our return he called and, with some surprise in his voice, told me, "Guess what? My vitamin D3 level was undetectable." He immediately began taking 50,000 IU per week for twelve weeks and now takes 2,000–4,000 IU every day.

Vitamin D, also called the sunshine vitamin, is the latest hot new thing in medicine. This once staid substance is suddenly at the center of a large amount of speculation and research. There have been many intriguing results of studies linking a vitamin D3 deficiency to a great variety of illnesses, from depression to cancer—although as yet there is very little causual evidence. Conversely, it may also offer protection from a range of other illnesses from the flu to heart disease. Many doctors now recommend that their patients—especially those patients at high risk for a deficiency, including women at menopause; dark-skinned, veiled women; people with multiple fractures; pregnant or breast-feeding women; and those with inflammatory bowel disease and celiac disease—be screened by a blood test periodically for blood levels of vitamin D3, although there is no consensus on what a normal range should be. While almost everyone understands the importance of getting his or her daily vitamins to maintain good health, very few people actually know what a vitamin is. Vitamins have literally shaped history. For hundreds of years exploration was limited by the existence of a deadly disease known as scurvy. Scurvy is a disease characterized by vitamin C deficiency. Vitamin C is necessary for collagen synthesis in humans. Severe deficiency leads to malaise, skin spots, bleeding

Screening for vitamin D deficiency recommended in individuals with multiple fractures, pregnant and breastfeeding women, dark-skinned individuals, veiled women, post-menopausal women, and patients with inflammatory bowel disease and celiac disease.

from mucus membranes, loss of teeth, and jaundice. It can be fatal. On long-distance voyages it killed passengers and crew members; in 1499 the legendary explorer Vasco da Gama lost 116 of his 170-man crew, and twenty years later 208 of Magellan's 230 men perished, almost all of them from a very strange disease. By 1614 doctors suspected scurvy was caused by a dietary deficiency, specifically the lack of an acid found in citrus fruit. In 1747 Scottish surgeon James Lind conducted the first clinical trial and proved that this disease could be treated and prevented by supplementing a diet with citrus fruits. The Royal Navy continued to insist that any acid would have the same result and as a result lost an estimated 130,000 enlisted sailors to disease during the Seven Years' War. Throughout the eighteenth century the navy lost more sailors to scurvy than in all battles combined. It wasn't until the Royal Navy added fresh lemons to the daily diet during the Napoleonic Wars that scurvy was finally eradicated.

In a similar advance, beginning in 1884 Japanese researchers successfully eliminated beriberi from the Japanese navy by adding larger amounts of meat, barley, and fruit to their sailors' normal diet. Beriberi is caused by nutritional deficiency of vitamin B1 (thiamine). Severe deficiency leads to weight loss, neuropathy, heart failure, and death.

But the basic principle of vitamins had been established: Certain nutrients that are absolutely essential to maintain good health are not produced by the body and have to be gotten from some outside source. In 1905 British biochemist Sir Frederick Hopkins discovered that some of those nutrients necessary for normal growth and health are found in ordinary foods. It wasn't until 1912 that Polish biochemist Casimir Funk proposed the theory that a variety of diseases in addition to scurvy, including rickets and pellagra, could be prevented or cured by dietary supplements that he called "vita [life] amines," which he shortened to "vitamines." He gave them that name believing these substances were from a group of organic compounds known as amines, which means they are derived from ammonia——that contained nitrogen. Several years later, when it became clear that some of these substances didn't fit that definition he dropped the "e" and the word "vitamin" became firmly entrenched in our vocabulary.

The story of vitamin D began almost two centuries ago. In 1822, in Warsaw, Poland, physician Jedrzej Sniadeki noted with curiosity that the disease rickets was common in the smoky, polluted industrial city but occurred only rarely in rural agricultural areas. Rickets is a terrible disease that strikes mainly children; it results in a weakening of the bones and often leads to fractures and deformities, including bowed legs, spinal curvature, and enlarged wrists and ankle joints. Believing a lack of sunlight might be the cause of the disease he experimented with two groups of children and proved that exposure to the healing rays of the sun could prevent or cure the disease.

Eventually it was discovered that the protective agent produced by the body when sunlight touches skin was vitamin D3. A century later researchers in the United States and England proved that irradiated foods—foods that are exposed to radiation to kill bacteria and certain insects as a method of increasing shelf life that also increases the potency of natural vitamin D3—also provided protection from rickets in children and adolescents and a similar disease, osteomalacia, in adults. By fortifying—adding vitamin D3 to—milk and bread by irradiating it, developed nations had pretty much eliminated rickets by the end of the Roaring Twenties.

Ironically, it turns out that by the accepted definition technically vitamin D isn't really a vitamin: A vitamin is a chemical component found in food that is required by the body to initiate the normal function of a physiological process or processes. It's a substance necessary for good health that can prevent specific diseases and that the body can't produce naturally but can be gotten by eating specific foods. Without that dietary supplement the body can't function properly. What makes vitamin D unique is that years after it was classified as a vitamin it was discovered that—unlike all the other common vitamins—it also can be produced by exposure to ultraviolet light such as the sun, for example. In fact, it is possible to get all of the vitamin D that is needed from exposure to the sun, and so, since the body actually can produce vitamin D under the right circumstances, it isn't a true vitamin. By that definition vitamin D is a hormone, meaning it is a substance produced by an organ—in this case, the skin—that travels throughout the bloodstream and has physiological effects on other organs or tissues. To settle matters, in 1971 it was reclassified in scientific terminology as "vitamin D3 hormone."

Whatever you call it, you need it. And you need a substantial amount of it. Once it is ingested or produced by the skin, the liver and kidneys convert it into its active form. Just about every type of tissue or organ in the human body—including bones, muscles, heart cells, brain cells, and fatty tissue—requires vitamin D to function optimally. Vitamin D also appears to regulate the genes that control cell growth and development, immune function, and metabolic control. In other words, vitamin D has an effect on just about all of the systems of the body.

Vitamin D3 is certainly one of the most underrated and least understood nutrients in the health and fitness world. We have a good understanding of exactly how this substance works once it gets into the body: After being metabolized (i.e., transformed into a chemical substance that can be used by the body), it helps regulate several functions, especially the absorption of calcium and phosphorous. It is an essential substance: Having too little vitamin D available to the organs and tissues that need it throws the entire system out of whack. The problem is that we don't yet understand the effect of vitamin D deficiency in many conditions. What we do know, and what has come to intrigue scientists and researchers, is that often when many serious diseases are diagnosed, vitamin D deficiency is among the many biochemical abnormalities present. But no one has yet been able to determine what role—if any—that deficiency plays in the disease. Do those conditions occur because of the lack of vitamin D, or is the lack of vitamin D the result of the disease? It's the old cause-or-effect conundrum.

The recognition of this connection between a vitamin D deficiency and numerous conditions is relatively recent in the industrialized world. One might assume that, unlike the citizens of Warsaw in 1822, most people have easy access to a diet that provides adequate vitamin D (fortified milk, cheese, fish) and could increase their vitamin D levels by spending significant time outdoors. The best source of vitamin D3 is sunlight, which is not owned, patented, trademarked, or in any other way controlled by any commercial entity. It's free and readily available. Because there is no opportunity for anyone to profit from sunlight there is little financial incentive for any company to do extensive research into its value in maintaining health. So until very recently there just hasn't been a lot of attention focused on this substance.

This is true of researchers and physicians as well as individuals. In 1999, Dr. Frank Domino, a professor of family medicine at the University of Massachusetts Medical School and the editor in chief of the medical textbook *The 5-Minute Clinical Consult,* began caring for a family that had moved to central Massachusetts from the North African nation of Sudan. As Dr. Domino remembers, "About two years after settling in the United States the oldest of the four children tore the ACL in his knee while playing soccer. Soon after, a second child suffered a broken leg, then the third child broke an arm. Within a year and a half all four children had fractured an arm or a leg. I became suspicious of child abuse or neglect and asked the parents to meet in my office. I knew something really was wrong when the father arrived with his arm in a cast. 'What happened?' I asked.

" 'I do not know,' he said. 'I just banged my arm on the mirror of a parked car.'

"I was concerned something very serious was going on. After consulting an endocrinologist I drew everyone's blood and tested for 25 hydroxy vitamin D levels. Each of their three sons had a very low level of vitamin D in their blood. But most concerning was their teenage daughter, whose vitamin D level was 'undetectable,' meaning she had no vitamin D. I immediately began prescribing large, regular doses of vitamin D.

"From this somewhat humbling experience, I learned about vitamin D metabolism, deficiency, and most importantly, how to diagnose and treat it. This family has remained in my practice, and not one of them has suffered an orthopedic injury since then."

It has long been known that by interacting with calcium, vitamin D3 helps build bone strength and healthy teeth. What's emerging is a very strong and growing body of evidence showing that it also might prevent or at least reduce the occurrence of many serious conditions and diseases. Investigators from the University of Pittsburgh Graduate School of Public Health, for example, compared blood samples from three thousand women who had normal pregnancies with samples from seven hundred women who eventually developed preeclampsia—a potentially very serious and even life-threatening disease. This study, published in 2013 in *Epidemiology*, found that during their first twenty-six weeks of pregnancy women with a vitamin D deficiency are 40 percent more likely to develop severe preeclampsia than women with adequate levels of this vitamin.

Other studies have associated a vitamin D deficiency during pregnancy with an array of potentially dangerous problems. A small Korean study done at Seoul's University School of Medicine and published in *American Journal of Obstetrics & Gynecology* in 2013 confirmed earlier studies by finding that 85 percent of pregnant women diagnosed with gestational diabetes had low levels of vitamin D and suggested that this deficiency may also lead to problems like low birth weight and development of weakened bones.

Unfortunately, a vitamin D deficiency is highly prevalent among children worldwide and can lead to a variety of serious medical issues. The 2013 Bogota School Children Cohort published in the *Pediatric Infectious Disease Journal* followed almost three thousand Colombian children of eight to nine years old for an entire school year. Most of these children came from medium-to-low-income families. Researchers reported,

Vitamin D,
together with calcium,
helps builds strong bones
and healthy teeth.

"Vitamin D deficient (VDD) children had higher rates of vomiting, diarrhea with vomiting (symptoms often present in children with acute viral and bacterial gastrointestinal infections) and earache or ear discharge with fever than Vitamin D sufficient children. . . . VDD children had twice as many days with diarrhea and vomiting. . . . These results add to the growing body of evidence supporting a role for Vitamin D in the susceptibility to infection related illness in children."

The first hint that a vitamin D deficiency could be related to the presence of a serious disease came from a statistical study published in 1941 by pathologist Frank Apperly, which demonstrated that the incidence of nonskin cancers in America increased as you moved north into the cooler latitudes where there was less year-round exposure to sunlight. So sunlight, Apperly decided, had to provide "a relative immunity to nonskin cancers."

In 1974, Frank Garland and his brother, epidemiologist Cedric F. Garland, were startled by a slide presentation made during a seminar at Johns Hopkins that showed people in the American North were dying of breast and colon cancer at almost twice the rate of people living in the Southwest. Nobody seemed to know why, although there was some speculation that barbecuing, eating other possibly carcinogenic foods, pollution, or other environmental factors possibly were responsible for this variance. Having just driven cross-country from San Diego to Baltimore, the Garland brothers suspected the availability of sunlight might account for that difference and began researching their theory. Six years later the *International Journal of Epidemiology* published their study noting that vitamin D was perhaps capable of markedly decreasing the risk of colon cancer. As Frank Garland

Four decades ago, people in northern North America were dying at twice the rate from breast and colon cancer as those living in the Southwest.

later remembered, their report created a stir, especially among people who accepted that the sun "was a dangerous cause of skin cancer and a peril to be avoided."

The Garland brothers spent their careers proving the strength of this link. A two-decade-long cohort study of Chicago residents demonstrated that people with the highest amount of vitamin D had half the incidence of colon cancer as those who had the lowest intake. This was the very first study to prove that vitamin D and calcium supplements reduced the risk of colon cancer. Other studies that they conducted reinforced these findings.

Many studies since then have almost universally supported the contention that a deficiency of vitamin D could be associated with an increase in the incidence of several common types of cancer—notably, prostate cancer. Prostate cancer is the most common form of cancer for men; more than 31,000 men die from it each year. In 1990, scientists speculated that a deficiency of vitamin D3 might actually be a primary cause or promoter of this disease. There was a substantial amount of statistical evidence to support that conclusion, in particular the odd fact that American men were almost ten times more likely to develop prostate cancer than Japanese men, whose diet is rich in fatty fish oil, which has high levels of vitamin D.

Among the leading researchers was epidemiologist Gary Schwartz, from Wake Forest University, who mirrored the work done by the Garland brothers and provided indisputable statistical evidence proving that men who spent more time in the sun were less likely to be diagnosed with prostate cancer. In addition, Dr. Schwartz discovered an intriguing correlation between death rates from prostate cancer and multiple sclerosis, which also is known to be associated with a lack of exposure to sunlight.

Schwartz acknowledges he did not become a scientist to pursue the causes of cancer, explaining, "In my previous life I was a primate biologist. I was interested in the evolution of monkeys, including the evolution of pigment and color. While I was excited about it, I eventually discovered that it was an area in which you can spend your entire career figuring out why an animal evolved in a specific way and when you're finished there are seven people who are interested in it. But if you can figure out why certain diseases are common to certain groups and if you can solve that problem—which is intellectually no different than the animal studies—then 70,000 people are interested in the results."

That realization changed his future plans, and after obtaining his PhD, Schwartz returned to school for a second degree, this one in epidemiology. "I didn't even know where the prostate was located when I started my research. The only reason I focused on that was because my advisor suggested I look at prostate cancer. And when I did I was struck by how little was known for certain about this disease." Among the many interesting facts that Schwartz discovered was that African Americans are proportionally far more likely to be diagnosed with prostate cancer and to die from it than Caucasians: 2.4 times more likely to die from it, in fact. It occurred to him that another disease that is more common among African Americans than Caucasians is rickets. "It's well-known that rickets can be caused by a lack of exposure to sunlight and [that] individuals with darker skin were at greater risk for that disease because the melanin that gives skin its color also prevents the skin from absorbing ultraviolet light, making it difficult for them to produce vitamin D3. I thought, this might be simple-minded, but if Blacks are at risk for one disease that's understood to be caused by a vitamin D3 deficiency, why couldn't they be at risk for another disease for the same reason? I wondered if I could develop a rickets-based model for vitamin D3 deficiency for prostate cancer."

The same type of data that had sparked the curiosity of the Garland brothers almost two decades earlier fascinated Schwartz. He began by comparing mortality rates for prostate cancer in each of the 3,073 counties in the United States with the amount of ultraviolet radiation that fell on each county and discovered "[a] striking inverse mortality rate in Caucasians—because that was the only data available—and the amount of ultraviolet radiation. It turned out the farther north you go the less sunlight and more prostate cancer you find. There is more prostate cancer in Maine than in Boston; but more in Boston than there is in Virginia, and it remains true all the way down to Florida."

As it has long been accepted that spending too much time in the sun can cause cancer, Schwartz's contention that spending time in the sun actually can prevent cancer was practically ridiculed. As he remembers, "A lot of people tried to talk me out of this research, believing it was so far-fetched it might hurt my career. They thought they were doing me a favor. At a conference in the mid-1990s, for example, I remember hearing a group of well-known oncologists discussing prostate cancer and one of them slapped his leg, literally slapped his leg, then laughed out loud and said, 'No, wait, wait. I know what it is. It's sunlight!' And they all laughed at that thought. I guess I didn't blame them, it seemed pretty outrageous that a researcher nobody ever heard of could discover this link."

The farther north one lives, the less one gets sunlight, and, tragically, the more one gets prostate cancer.

The punch line changed completely in 1998 when Schwartz and his team proved that prostate cell lines could indeed activate vitamin D3. Following the initial observation, "We did quite a lot of experimentation with vitamin D3 and prostate cells. For a long time people had difficulty accepting this thesis—until we actually discovered that the prostate can synthesize the active form of vitamin D3. If the prostate manufactures its own vitamin D3 it's obvious that it must need it.

"I got so excited about all this that I became a bit of a caricature. Even I began wondering if I had gone too far when I discovered a little yellow sticky that someone had left on my car on which they had written, 'Go ahead, just ask me about vitamin D3.'"

Since Schwartz's discovery extensive research has reinforced his conclusion. In 2001, for example, researchers at England's Keele University School of Medicine published three different studies showing a provable link among exposure to ultraviolet light, skin type, and prostate cancer, reporting that men who spent extensive time in the sun, whether for recreation or by occupation, reduced their risk of being diagnosed with prostate cancer. Eventually the concept that spending time in the sun can reduce chances of cancer—and, in fact, several different types of cancer—became an accepted fact. As the *Journal of the National Cancer Institute* reported in 2006, "Among Caucasians in the United States cancer mortality for several prominent cancers, including cancer of the breast, prostate and colon, shows a striking latitudinal gradient, with increased mortality rates among those individuals residing in the northern states compared with individuals residing in southern states. These patterns persist even after confounding variables like socioeconomic status, urban and residual residence, Hispanic heritage and other risk factors are taken into account."

Other studies have continued to suggest that vitamin D3 is likely a strong weapon against prostate cancer. In 2014 the *Clinical Cancer Research* journal published a study that showed a strong connection between low blood levels of the vitamin and aggressive prostate cancer, a link that was especially strong in African American men. However, this same study also showed that very high levels of vitamin D actually increased the risk of prostate cancer.

At a 2004 NIH conference on vitamin D and cancer, researchers announced the results of the first human interventional trial—a study in which an observed behavior is changed and the results of that change can be measured. Investigators from the University of Toronto found that 2,000 international units of vitamin D3 taken daily reduced or prevented increases in the PSA of men diagnosed with prostate cancer. PSA is the measurement of protein in the prostate, and elevated levels may indicate the presence of prostate cancer. This study suggested that perhaps vitamin D3 had a measurable impact in fighting—and even possibly preventing—prostate cancer.

While the results of these studies have consistently shown the value of vitamin D in fighting prostate cancer, the mystery of why that is true has yet to be solved. A 2014 study conducted by researchers at the University of Colorado Cancer Center and published in the online journal *Prostate* stated, "When you take vitamin D and put it on prostate cancer cells, it inhibits their growth. . . . We wanted to understand what genes vitamin D is turning on or off in prostate cancer." Their study suggests that vitamin D might impact prostate cancer by upregulating a specific gene that works to suppress inflammation, which "is thought to drive many cancers including prostate, gastric and colon."

As some researchers had suspected, in addition to colon and prostate cancer, the presence—or deficiency—of vitamin D has been shown to have a direct impact on the risk of being diagnosed with several different types of cancer, including bladder, uterine, esophageal, rectal, ovarian, and especially breast cancer. Frank Garland published two studies in 1989 and 1990, for example, that showed a direct connection between a vitamin D deficiency and breast cancer. Studies published in 2005 and 2006 by researchers at the University of California at San Diego's Moores Cancer Center used a World Health Organization database that tracked the incidence, mortality, and prevalence of cancer in 175 countries to show "a clear association between a deficiency in exposure to sunlight [vitamin D]" and ovarian and kidney cancer.

A 2006 report in that same issue of the *NCI Journal* cited two epidemiological studies, which studied almost seven thousand participants and suggested "sunlight may reduce the risk of non-Hodgkins lymphoma and may be associated with increased survival rates in patients with early stage melanoma." That was confirmed in 2007, when researchers at Germany's Johannes-Gutenberg University reported their findings in the *International Journal of Cancer*: a "reduced overall lymphoma risk among subjects having spent vacations in sunny climates or frequently used sun beds or sunlamps." In other words, exposure to UV rays statistically reduced the occurrence of cancers of the lymphatic system.

In addition to reducing the risk of being diagnosed with these cancers, there is evidence that vitamin D may help patients survive it. A study of more than one thousand colon

A 2006 study:
Sunlight may reduce
the risk of non-Hodgkin's
lymphoma.

cancer patients being treated at Boston's Dana-Farber Cancer Institute showed that patients with high levels of vitamin D3 were twice as likely to survive as those patients with low levels. A similar British study found that skin cancer patients with low levels of vitamin D3 had more than a 33 percent chance of relapsing than those people with high levels.

While the statistical evidence from numerous studies makes a very strong association between low levels of vitamin D and increased risks of prostate, colon, and other cancers, it is important to note that the ability of sunlight or UV rays to protect against cancer hasn't been proven definitively in clinical trials. Dr. Ronald Lieberman, program director of the Prostate and Urologic Cancer Research Group at the National Cancer Institute Division of Cancer Prevention admitted, "We don't have a bit of evidence that I could show you to say it will work as a preventative." But in addition to the growing mountain of data that makes a strong case, he does add that clinical studies have suggested that vitamin D3 will augment the effects of chemotherapy or radiation on the system.

If the benefits of vitamin D were limited to its impact on cancer, that alone would be sufficient to make sure we were all getting enough of it. But, for thus far inexplicable reasons, vitamin D appears to offer additional protections against other very serious diseases. Heart disease, for example, is the most common cause of death for American men. And researchers at the Harvard School of Public Health and Brigham and Women's Hospital made an association between heart disease and a vitamin D deficiency in a study that tracked almost fifty thousand health professionals for ten years. During that period slightly fewer than five hundred of the men had suffered a heart attack or died of heart disease. The report concluded that men with a vitamin D3 deficiency had twice the chance of having a heart attack as men with adequate D3 levels. The author of this study, Dr. Edward Giovannucci, emphasized that—as in so many other reports—no one yet knows how or why vitamin D3 appears to offer this protection, although he suggests it might lower blood pressure, reduce inflammation, and perhaps even reduce calcification of the arteries.

Austrian researchers at the University of Graz measured vitamin D3 levels in 3,200 patients averaging sixty years old then tracked them for eight years. During that period 463 of that group died of heart disease—and 307 of them had low levels of vitamin D. The authors emphasized that the study "could not determine a causal link for mortality."

A Harvard Medical School study published in *Circulation* in 2008 tracked 1,700 people over fifty-nine years old for seven years and found that those people with a vitamin D deficiency had twice the risk of heart attack, heart failure, and stroke as healthy participants. Once again, though, the lead researcher, in this case Dr. Thomas Wang, could not make a definitive statement, instead pointing out, "What hasn't been proven yet is that vitamin D deficiency actually causes increased risk of cardiovascular disease."

A 2009 study reported by the Intermountain Medical Center in Salt Lake reached a similar conclusion. Twenty-eight thousand participants had been tracked for two years and at the end of that brief period those patients with the lowest vitamin D3 levels were 77 percent more likely to have died or suffered a stroke and almost half were more likely to have developed coronary artery disease than those participants who maintained normal levels.

But "the most comprehensive epidemiological study ever

Although not proven,
vitamin D deficiency may
predispose one to increased
risk of heart attacks
and stroke.

conducted of the association between vitamin D and mortality has revealed that low vitamin D levels are directly linked to early death from heart disease and other causes." The Copenhagen City Heart Study, which concluded in 2012, followed more than ten thousand men and women for three decades and monitored all their health developments. During that time period 6,747 participants died, and according to researchers, "There was a huge disparity in disease and death rates among those in the low Vitamin D group compared to those in the high Vitamin D group. . . . Most striking was the finding that those with the lowest levels of Vitamin D were 81 percent more likely to die from ischemic heart disease or myocardial infarction [heart attack]." To confirm these startling results the researchers looked at seventeen other similar studies and found that "[d]ecreased levels of Vitamin D were found to be directly associated with a higher risk of disease and death in virtually every study," according to study author Dr. Borge G. Nordestgaard.

Further evidence of this connection was presented in 2014 at the American College of Cardiology's annual Scientific Session in which researchers reported that more than 70 percent of patients undergoing coronary angiography, an imaging process done in patients with some symptoms of heart disease, had a vitamin D deficiency.

Among the primary causes of heart disease is high blood pressure, and a 2014 study published online in the *Lancet Diabetes & Endocrinology* reported that low levels of vitamin D have been shown to have a direct association with high blood pressure. In fact, other studies have shown that vitamin D supplementation actually may be more effective at lowering blood pressure than restricting salt intake. A meta-analysis conducted by researchers from ten European nations, America, and Australia analyzed data from thirty-five studies involving more than 155,000 men and women of European descent and concluded that for each 10 percent increase in vitamin D levels there was a corresponding 8.1 percent decrease in the risk of developing high blood pressure. As the study leader, University of South Australia Professor Elina Hypponen, said, "In view of the costs and side effects associated with antihypertensive (high blood pressure) drugs, the potential to prevent or reduce blood pressure and therefore the risk of hypertension with vitamin D is very attractive." As the lead author of the study, Dr. Karani S. Vimaleswaran, told the audience at the 2013 European Human Genetics Conference, "Our study strongly suggests that some cases of cardiovascular disease could be prevented through vitamin D supplements or food fortification."

The Garland brothers' initial observation that the incidence of colon cancer has a direct correlation to available sunlight also has been applied to several other serious diseases, including metabolic conditions. There is evidence that vitamin D may play a role in type 1 diabetes. A thirty-year Finnish study that followed ten thousand children from birth showed that a child growing up in Finland, with its limited exposure to the sun, is about four hundred times more likely to develop type 1 diabetes than a Venezuelan child, who lives in year-round sunlight. For some thus far unexplained reason Finland has the highest incidence of type 1 diabetes in the world; but this 2003 study reported that the children who consistently received vitamin D supplements during their early years reduced the risk of eventually being diagnosed with type 1 diabetes by almost 90 percent.

Those astonishing results were supported by a 2013 Harvard School of Public Health study. Researchers found that "[h]aving adequate levels of vitamin D during young adulthood may reduce the risk of adult-onset diabetes by as much as 50%." The lead author of the study, Kassandra Munger, noted, "It is surprising that a serious disease such as type 1 diabetes could perhaps be prevented by a simple and safe intervention."

Researchers from Tufts University and Tufts Medical School found that vitamin D also can help prevent type 2 diabetes. Their study, published by the American Diabetes Association journal *Diabetes Care* in 2012, analyzed blood taken from more than two thousand participants over two and a half years and found that "for every 5 nanogram per milliliter increase in Vitamin D, there was a 13% decrease in the risk of progression to diabetes." In the third of the cohort at most risk for diabetes because of skin color or other factors, those participants with the highest levels of vitamin D reduced their risk of being diagnosed with type 2 diabetes by 39 percent. According to Dr. Anastassios Pittas, codirector of the study, "Although there are well-recognized differences in vitamin D metabolism among different racial and ethnic groups, higher vitamin D status appears to be associated with lower risk of diabetes among all people regardless of skin color."

As with other diseases, there is considerable speculation about why vitamin D appears to have this dramatic effect in relation to type 2 diabetes. According to Dr. Pittas, previous studies have found vitamin D improves the ability of the pancreas to produce insulin. Insulin helps the body to use or store the glucose it gets from food. With less insulin resistance, individuals are less likely to develop type 2 diabetes.

Obesity has been shown to be a significant factor leading to diabetes, and numerous studies have proven there is a strong link between obesity and vitamin D deficiency. But here, some studies have indicated that obesity is the cause of the deficiency, rather than a lack of vitamin D leading to weight gain. While vitamin D doesn't appear to prevent or reduce obesity, a deficiency in obese people may be one of the reasons obesity leads so often to type 2 diabetes.

Vitamin D levels also seem to play a yet unknown role in several neurological diseases. For example, multiple sclerosis (MS), a disease in which an individual's own immune system attacks his or her central nervous system, occurs more frequently far north and far south of the equator than in climates bathed year-round in sunlight. As long ago as 1974 the *Journal of Environmental Studies* published the results of a small study that hinted that environmental factors, especially available sunlight, might trigger MS in genetically susceptible people. Since then several other international studies have supported that theory, but only recently has serious research begun. For example, according to the authors of a 2006 Harvard School of Public Health study published in *JAMA*, "The change in MS risk with migration among people of common ancestry strongly supports a role for environmental factors. One potential factor may be vitamin D exposure." Researchers in this large prospective study examined the medical records of more than eight million active-duty military members collected since the early 1980s and concluded, "Our results converge with a growing body of evidence supporting a protective role for vitamin D in MS development. Vitamin D is a potent immunomodulator."

Intrigued by these results, the NIH currently is supporting several studies focusing on the link between low levels of vitamin D and both the initial flare-up and relapsing episodes of MS symptoms.

Many people don't realize that several of the most common cognitive impairments are considered neurological disorders, including Alzheimer's and other forms of dementia, and that all of them may be affected by low vitamin D levels. A 2010 University of Exeter study published in the *Archives of Internal Medicine* followed 858 elderly adults and reported that during the six-year study those people with the lowest blood levels of vitamin D were 60 percent more likely to show signs of general cognitive decline and 31 percent more likely to show declines in their ability to plan, organize, and prioritize (executive functioning) than those people with sufficient blood levels of vitamin D.

A University of California at San Diego Medical School study presented at the 2014 Acute Cardiovascular Care meeting analyzed data from eight international studies in which 26,000 patients between the ages of fifty and seventy-nine were followed for sixteen years. In addition to finding a link between patients with low levels of vitamin D and death from cardiovascular disease they also noted something unexpected: There was a significant link between vitamin D levels and the neurological outcome in people who suffered life-threatening heart attacks. Researchers analyzed fifty-three unconscious patients who had been resuscitated following cardiac arrest at Seoul Hospital in Korea—in each instance their heart had stopped pumping blood, meaning their brain was deprived of oxygen for a period of time. Six months after cardiac arrest 65 percent of patients with a vitamin D deficiency had a "poor neurological outcome" compared with 23 percent

There appears to be
a link between vitamin D
deficiency and
Alzheimer's dementia.

who had a normal range of vitamin D in their system. In fact, by that time 29 percent of vitamin D–deficient patients had died, while all of the patients with normal vitamin D levels had survived.

Researchers in Qatar wondered if vitamin D levels might be associated with a diagnosis of attention deficit hyperactive disorder (ADHD). They recruited slightly more than twenty-five hundred school-age children split equally between those with ADHD and those without this disorder and found that the average level of vitamin D was about 15 percent lower in children with this learning problem than those without it, showing, according to the report, "Vitamin D deficiency was greater among children . . . with the diagnosis of ADHD compared to controls."

While this and other studies have shown a correlation between low levels of vitamin D and impaired brain function, the reasons for the correlation remain elusive. Laboratory studies have shown that vitamin D appears to be able to clear Alzheimer-causing plaque in the brain: researchers working at the University of California reported in the *Journal of Alzheimer's Disease* in 2012 that they had "identified the intracellular mechanisms regulated by vitamin D3 that may help the body clear the brain of amyloid beta, the main component of plaques associated with Alzheimer's disease. The early findings show that vitamin D3 may activate key genes and cellular signaling networks to help stimulate the immune system to clear the amyloid-beta protein." According to the author of the study, Dr. Mathew T. Mizwicki from the University of California at Riverside, this Alzheimer's Association–funded study "demonstrates that active forms of vitamin D3 may be an important regulator of immune activities of macrophages in helping to clear amyloid plaques by directly regulating the expression of genes, as well as the structural physical workings of the cells."

As America's population ages, Alzheimer's and other forms of dementia are beginning to strain our existing facilities, and considerable research is being done to discover the cause and possible ways to prevent or cure these disorders. The role played by vitamin D is becoming increasingly important. Scientists have found vitamin D receptors, which are rarely found in places in the body where they are not used, in the brain. They also have found the enzymes needed to process vitamin D, which suggest an association without being able to provide an explanation. In a study published in the journal *Neurology* in August 2014, researchers at the University of Exeter Medical School examined data from sixteen hundred participants in the U.S. Cardiovascular Health Study compiled over a seven-year period. This was the largest study thus far conducted to examine the association between a vitamin D deficiency and dementia and, according to Keith Fargo, director of scientific programs for the Alzheimer's Association, showed "[t]here is a link between vitamin D and the development of Alzheimer's." Participants with moderately low levels of vitamin D were 1.7 times more likely to develop some form of dementia than individuals with normal levels, while those people with severely low levels had more than double the risk—2.2 times—of eventually developing some form of dementia compared with those people having acceptable levels of vitamin D in their blood.

Another 2014 study, this one published in the *Journal of Clinical Endocrinology and Metabolism*, examined nineteen good studies and concluded that people with a vitamin D deficiency were twice as likely as those with normal levels to eventually be diagnosed with the brain disorder schizophrenia.

Based on these and similar neurological studies it was not surprising that two French studies, with about two thousand participants, published in *Annals of Nutrition and Metabolism* found that "dietary vitamin D intake was significantly and positively related to short-term memory." Participants filed regular reports over the course of the study, and researchers followed up with them thirteen years later. While they reported a strong association between levels of vitamin D and short-term memory, defined as the storage of information, they failed to find that association between vitamin D intake and declarative memory, which is the ability to recall facts and events.

For many reasons a low level of vitamin D makes more of an impact on older people. A Dutch study showed that, in addition to impacting brain function, vitamin D shared a connection to physical performance in older people. More than two thousand men and women over fifty-five were tested on their ability to perform a variety of simple, daily tasks, including walking up and down a staircase, rising from a chair, and cutting their toenails. Their blood levels were then measured and correlated against the results of physical tests. As reported in 2013 by the *Journal of Clinical Endocrinology and Metabolism*, a measureable vitamin D deficiency "was associated with an increased number of disabilities."

That obviously makes sense, as the importance of vitamin D to building and maintaining strong bones was first recognized almost two centuries ago. It has become an essential tool in the fight to prevent osteoporosis, a common disease in which reduced bone density often leads to easily fractured bones and other complications. A primary cause of osteo-porosis is a reduced level of calcium in bones, and among the many properties of vitamin D is its ability to help the body absorb calcium. While there is no evidence that vitamin D can reverse osteoporosis once someone is diagnosed with it, what it can do in many instances is mitigate the potential damage.

According to the International Osteoporosis Founda-tion, "Vitamin D is important for bone and muscle develop-ment, function and preservation. For this reason it is a vital component in the maintenance of bone strength and in the prevention of falls and osteoporotic fractures." In addition, the foundation claims that "[p]reventing vitamin D deficiency has a major impact on falls and osteoporotic fractures. . . . Vitamin D affects fracture risk through its effect on bone metabolism and on falls risk." A 2014 Cochrane review— Cochrane reviews are well-respected summaries of properly conducted studies—of fifty-three recent studies reported that vitamin D supplements containing calcium were espe-cially effective in preventing fractures, including far-too-common hip fractures. However, it is important to note that recent data have shown that taking more than seven hundred milligrams of calcium daily does not improve bone mineral density or lower the risk of fracture—and it also may in-crease the risk of cardiovascular events. That isn't true of vi-tamin D: A 2009 analysis of more than forty thousand elderly people found that taking vitamin D daily "reduced hip and non-spine fractures by 20 percent," while a companion study showed it reduced falls by 19 percent. Hip fractures are a ma-jor health problem in the United States and throughout the world. In 2003, more than three hundred thousand individuals were hospitalized with hip fractures in the United States. Hip fractures substantially increase the risk of major morbidity and of death in the elderly.

Certainly one aspect of physical performance that has become a matter of medical concern is erectile dysfunction, one of the most common problems among American men. While there has been voluminous research into the causes of this sexual problem, and there are several known causes as well as effective treatments, a 2014 study published in the *Journal of Sexual Medicine* reported that men diagnosed with severe erectile dysfunction were significantly more vitamin D deficient than men with mild sexual problems.

In women, at least one study has shown that a low level of vitamin D can increase the risk of being diagnosed with uterine fibroids—benign but often painful tumors in the uterus—and too often result in hysterectomies. In 2013 *Epidemiology* reported an NIH study of more than one thousand women whose health status was compared with their vitamin D levels and blood tests. Two-thirds of participants reported having fibroid tumors. Researchers concluded that women with acceptable levels of vitamin D decreased their risk for being diagnosed with fibroids by 32 percent and that each 10 percent increase in the presence of vitamin D in blood resulted in a 20 percent lowered risk. The lead author of this study, epidemiologist Donna Baird, kept it in perspective, explaining, "[s]ufficient levels of vitamin D are probably good for several health outcomes, and fibroids may be one of them."

Of all the illnesses speculatively related to sunlight, none is more common than respiratory diseases like cold and flu. Throughout history people tend to get colds when it gets cold, and most of them reach the obvious conclusion: I got sick because I went outside without proper protection. There may well be a lot of evidence to support that conclusion, but now there is also some belief that an immune system weakened by a lack of vitamin D may contribute to it. For decades people have insisted that vitamin C is the best way to prevent or treat colds and flu, but a growing body of evidence hints strongly that protection might be much greater with the sunshine vitamin. The theory that a lack of vitamin D from sunlight can act as a trigger to these common diseases was initially proposed in 1981, but it is only recently that serious studies have been conducted. While some studies have shown little or no benefit to be gained from vitamin D supplements taken during periods of reduced sunlight, other studies have produced intriguing results. A 2013 Japanese double-blind, randomized, and fully controlled study with 354 participants published in the *American Journal of Clinical Nutrition* concluded that vitamin D actually was far more successful in fighting colds or flu than the most popular antiviral drugs available. Initially, the children taking vitamin D became ill at the same rate as those children in the control group. But after a month, as the level of vitamin D in the children's blood peaked, the protective effects of this vitamin became clear. Compared with those who received popular remedies, whose risk was reduced by less than 10 percent, children receiving 1,200 IU of vitamin D daily who had been exposed to infection reduced their risk of eventually being diagnosed with a cold or flu by 50 percent or greater. Overall, children receiving vitamin D had a 40 percent lower chance of getting the most common type of flu than the control group.

The largest study done so far, conducted by University of Colorado, Denver, Division of Emergency Medicine and published by *Archives of Internal Medicine* in 2009, analyzed data from nineteen thousand adults and adolescents gathered over a six-year span. Researchers found that people with low levels of vitamin D were 36 percent more likely to suffer from a respiratory infection than people with normal or high levels in their system. As Dr. Adit Ginde, a director of the study, comments, "The findings of our study support an important role for vitamin D in prevention of common respiratory infections, such as colds and the flu."

Researchers have begun looking into associated areas where vitamin D levels might have a real difference. The fact that vitamin D appears to provide at least some protection against colds, flu, and upper respiratory infections has led scientists to find out if it is useful in fighting diseases like tuberculosis, which affect the respiratory system. Years ago, long before the availability of antibiotics, the standard treatment for TB was sunlight and sun lamps. In fact, many of the early settlers in the Southwest moved there because its dry, sunny climate offered some respite from the disease, without the oppressive heat in the pre-air-conditioned South.

Without doubt there is at least a tenuous connection between a vitamin D deficiency and tuberculosis. As Indian researchers reported in 2013, citing several small studies, "Strong data is emerging for active tuberculosis in Vitamin D deficiency subjects." A 2013 British study that examined the incidence of tuberculosis in the city of Birmingham over almost three decades found "strong evidence for seasonality. . . . Winter dips in sunshine correlated with peaks in tuberculosis incidence six months later." An Indian study published in the *World Journal of Pharmacy and Pharmaceutical Sciences* in early 2014 compared vitamin D levels in slightly more than five hundred patients diagnosed with TB and a similar number of people without the disease and concluded, "After adjustment of confounding factors of Vitamin D, (including cigarette smoking, climate and diet) it was clearly demonstrated that all patients of tuberculosis had low level of vitamin D in blood."

Tuberculosis is more common in certain parts of the world because of climate, diet, and lack of sanitary facilities, and it is estimated that more than a million and a half people die from it each year. A 2013 clinical study conducted by the Ojha Institute of Chest Disease in Karachi, Pakistan, randomized 259 patients diagnosed with TB. Half of the group received large doses of vitamin D while the other half received a placebo. While somewhat similar studies have not demonstrated dramatic results, in this study researchers concluded that "high dose vitamin D supplementation can lead to a more marked clinical and radiological recovery in all patients with pulmonary TB and boost host immune responses in patients deficient in vitamin D."

And finally there is the biggest unanswered question: Does a vitamin D deficiency have a measureable effect on mortality? Does vitamin D help us live longer? Certainly the most tantalizing study, published in 2008 in *Archives of Internal Medicine,* stated flatly that people with a "vitamin D3 deficiency are as much as twice as likely to die, compared to people whose blood contains higher amounts of the sunshine vitamin." While that seems like an incredible conclusion to reach, a study conducted by researchers at the Medical University of Graz, Austria, gathered blood samples of thirty-two hundred people with an average age of sixty-two scheduled for a heart examination. Eight years later 463 of those patients had died—

and 307 of them had low levels of vitamin D3. The authors emphasized, as most studies do, that this "study could not determine a causal link for mortality."

That result was confirmed in a large 2009 study reported by the International Medical Center in Salt Lake City. About twenty-eight thousand participants were divided into three groups and tracked for two years. During that time those people with the lowest vitamin D3 levels were 77 percent more likely to have died or suffered a stroke, and almost half were more likely to have developed coronary artery disease than those people maintaining normal levels of vitamin D3.

One of the largest studies of vitamin D and mortality rates, which compared the blood levels of vitamin D to premature death, included 566,583 participants from fourteen countries who were an average of fifty-five years old. It was done at the University of California at San Diego, and published by the *American Journal of Public Health* in 2014. In this systemic review of thirty-two studies, researchers found that people with low levels of vitamin D in the blood were twice as likely to die prematurely as those participants with normal or higher levels. Obviously it is possible there are many other reasons for this pretty astonishing result, and there have been other studies that do not support this conclusion; a 2014 Cochrane review of fifty trials that included 94,138 participants, for example, found that "[v]itamin D3 seems to decrease mortality in predominantly elderly women who are mainly in institutions and dependent care," whereas vitamin D2 had no effect on mortality. But these studies certainly should be strong enough to encourage people to maintain healthy levels of vitamin D in their system.

A Danish study published in *BMJ* in 2014 was especially

A 2008 study:
Individuals with vitamin D3
deficiency more likely to
die than those with
higher blood
vitamin D3 levels.

interesting because of its geographic location, since Danes are exposed to limited annual sunlight. Researchers at Copenhagen University Hospital analyzed data from ninety-six thousand people followed for as long as four decades and reported that those participants with chronically low levels of vitamin D had a 30 percent higher mortality rate and, not surprisingly, were 40 percent more likely to get tumorous growths.

And perhaps the largest study, also published in *BMJ* in 2014, examined the link between vitamin D levels and all-cause mortality, including cancer and heart disease. Researchers at the Department of Public Health and Primary Care at Cambridge University conducted a systematic review and meta-analysis of data from almost one hundred studies, including twenty-two clinically randomized, controlled trials, which included almost nine hundred thousand participants and concluded that "[s]upplementation with vitamin D3 significantly reduces overall mortality among older adults," although it is noted that more studies need to be done to determine the optimal dose and whether two forms of the vitamin, D2 and D3, lead to different outcomes.

Clearly there is ample evidence to support the fact that a deficiency of vitamin D can be associated with a host of medical conditions. It is estimated that about 25 percent of Americans have an insufficient amount of vitamin D to maintain good health, while another 39 percent are deficient. In 2006 researchers at the Mayo Clinic warned that too many people around the world are not getting enough vitamin D, describing this as "a largely unrecognized epidemic in many populations worldwide."

With vitamin D as easy to get as walking outside in the

sunlight, why are so many people deficient in it? First, there are many people who simply don't spend enough time in the sun. Ironically, the long campaign to prevent skin cancer, which is caused by overexposure to the sun, has been tremendously successful in convincing people either to reduce their exposure to the sun or to cover their exposed skin with highly effective sunscreen. But an unintended result of that campaign has been a substantial increase in the number of people diagnosed with a vitamin D deficiency, as sunblock not only blocks the sun but also prevents the skin from getting the UV rays it needs to produce vitamin D.

Geography also plays an important role, as the Garland brothers and Schwartz demonstrated; the farther away someone lives from the equator the more difficult it is for that person to get sufficient exposure to the sun—no matter how much time they might spend outside. In areas of the United States above the Mason-Dixon and in Canada, for example, there just isn't enough overhead sunlight from November through March to produce the ultraviolet rays to produce the desired levels of vitamin D—especially if people are wearing protective clothing to keep themselves warm. The altitude at which someone lives also affects natural vitamin D production; as the sun is more intense on the top of a mountain than at ground level, people actually produce more vitamin D on top of a mountain than they will lying on a beach.

While it is also possible to get vitamin D from foods, which is why it was mistakenly classified as a vitamin, it's really difficult to get enough of it on a regular basis to fulfill the basic requirements. Many Americans—especially teenagers—have reduced significantly the amount of fortified foods they eat or drink, including milk. Ironically, eating too much of the wrong foods can lead to obesity, which as explained above seems to cause a vitamin D deficiency.

It also has a lot to do with each individual. Older people, for example, have a more difficult time producing ample amounts of vitamin D naturally as their skin thins and their metabolism slows. The natural ability to produce vitamin D is also dependent on skin color. The darker the skin, the more difficult it is to absorb the UV rays necessary to produce it; for that reason African Americans are more likely to be vitamin D deficient than Caucasians. Interestingly, that may be the reason a considerably higher percentage of black women suffer from uterine fibroids than lighter-skinned women.

Lifestyle choices can also cause a vitamin D deficiency. People who cover themselves with clothing to protect themselves from the sun, including veiled woman, may not get a tan or sunburn—but they also may not get sufficient sun exposure. People who spend a significant amount of time indoors, including seniors, nursing home residents, and sedentary and homebound individuals, probably will not get enough sun.

Pregnant women, patients with MS, individuals with a history of fractures, and people taking certain medications, especially Dilantin, which is used commonly to treat epilepsy and seizures, also are often deficient in vitamin D and need to make sure they keep a close watch on their vitamin D levels.

Unfortunately, it is not only possible to be vitamin D deficient and not know it, it's extremely common. Unlike other health problems, a deficiency of vitamin D isn't always obvious. There are no direct symptoms, although common complaints include overall tiredness and general aches and pains—which are also the symptoms of countless other problems. A severe deficiency can sometimes be the cause of bone pain and weakness, difficulty in getting around, increased blood pressure, depression, and frequent infections. But the only certain way to determine if you're deficient is with a blood test. Doctors will check your 25(OH)D level in the blood.

It gets a little more complicated. While the level of vitamin D present in your blood can be measured, unfortunately there is no specific level that is universally defined as the right amount. Studies have been all over the place as far as how much vitamin D3 is necessary to maintain optimum health. Because each individual's genetic makeup helps determine how vitamin D3 is produced and utilized in the body, it's difficult to know precisely what constitutes a deficiency. The amount of vitamin D present in your body is measured in either nanomoles per liter or nanograms per milliliter. According to the NIH, levels below 30 nmol/L are too low to maintain overall health, while levels above 125 nmol/L are generally too high. The NIH recommends, "[l]evels of 50 nmol/L or above are sufficient for most people."

Then how much vitamin D do you need on a daily basis? You need as much as you need, and for each person that number is different depending on all the variables previously mentioned. You really don't need that much; 100 IU a day is sufficient to prevent rickets, for example, and until recently that was the recommended daily allowance. The NIH recommends that 600 IU is enough for children and for adults until they reach seventy-one, at which time they need a minimum of 800 IU daily, with a maximum of 4,000 IU. In 2011 the American Academy of Pediatrics raised their recommend dose from 200 IU, suggesting, "[a]ll children should get 400 International Units a day within a few days of birth."

Many children do not appear to be getting enough vitamin D, causing Dr. Frank Domino to state, "I believe at this point there is sufficient reason to have all children taking 1,000 international units and all teenaged females 2,000 IU's per day."

So if you need it, where can you get it? The best place to get vitamin D is from the sun wherever and whenever that is possible. It was said a long time ago that "only mad dogs and Englishmen go out in the midday sun," but in fact your body will produce more vitamin D in the middle of a sunny day than at any other time. A simple rule is that the best time of day to produce vitamin D is when your shadow is shorter than your height. While we all have heard the horror stories about people who have spent too much time in the sun, it is currently recommended that people in warmer climates spend twenty minutes a day in the summer and thirty minutes the rest of the year outside without sunscreen, and people with a darker complexion should consider an additional ten minutes. For a fair-skinned person, under perfect conditions your body is capable of producing somewhere between 10,000 and 25,000 IU of vitamin D in about the time it takes your skin to turn light pink. Here's a healthy hint: You produce the most vitamin D when you expose a larger area, your back for example, than areas like your limbs or face.

In those places too far from the equator to get sufficient sunlight in the winter months there are a lot of options. It is estimated that we can get as much as 20 percent of the vitamin D we need from certain foods, which include fortified milk, cheese, salmon, tuna, egg yolks, beef liver, herring, fortified breakfast cereals, orange juice, certain mushrooms, and fortified margarine. A tablespoon of cod liver oil contains 1,360 IU, more than twice as much as the next best thing, three ounces of swordfish, which contains 566 IU. From there the amount of vitamin D in food continues to diminish; a large egg, for example, contains only 41 IU, and even a cup of fortified orange juice contains fewer than 150 IU. It's important to remember that most often you won't be able to fulfill daily vitamin D needs just from your diet.

For that reason many people get their daily dose of vitamin D from supplements. It's important to be aware that both vitamin D2 and vitamin D3 are available in supplemental form. One can buy these from a pharmacy or a vitamin shop. It's generally agreed that D3 is likely more effective than D2 at replacing vitamin D in your system, but many studies of vitamin D2 are small and of short duration. The Vitamin D Council recommends D3, which is the type of vitamin D your body produces when exposed to the sun's UV rays. Vitamin D3 is synthesized from animal sources, while D2 is derived from plants. Epidemiologist Gary Schwartz points out, "The best source of Vitamin D3 still remains the sun—and it's free. My skin is so dark that I get tan just thinking about being in the sun. On very sunny days I use sunscreen. But I also take vitamin D3 supplements. They're safe and they're effective in reducing vitamin D3 deficiency, and I'll still get my vitamin D3 from the sun."

While vitamin D is completely safe when taken in sensible doses, there are some potential dangers. Some physicians caution patients against taking more than 4,000 IU daily, pointing out it is usually not needed and large doses increase the amount of calcium, which can be problematic in certain situations. The Vitamin D Council cautions against adults taking more than 10,000 IU without medical supervision.

Vitamin D toxicity, which can be harmful, is extremely rare. It generally requires massive doses. People who take as much as 4,000 IU a day are not in danger of overdosing on vitamin D.

There are people with certain conditions who need to be cautious about using vitamin D supplements. These include patients with tuberculosis, sarcoidosis, lymphoma, and a history of kidney stones. People with high blood calcium levels should consult their physician before supplementing vitamin D intake, and there are some medicines and medical conditions, including atrial fibrillation, Hodgkin's lymphoma, and kidney and liver disease, that can be adversely affected by the presence of too much vitamin D.

The mystery of vitamin D is slowly being unraveled. There is still so much about it that we don't know or don't understand. One of the major studies currently in progress will assess the efficacy of vitamin D supplementation compared with fish oil and a placebo. According to Dr. JoAnn Manson, a professor at Harvard Medical School, the principal investigator of the VITamin D and OmegA-3 TriaL (VITAL), it has been designed to provide evidence "to inform individual decisions, clinical recommendations, and public health guidelines about the use of vitamin D and marine omega-3 fatty acid supplements for the primary prevention of cancer and cardiovascular disease." Twenty thousand participants from all fifty states are in the process of being tracked for five years, and at the end of that time we will have a scientific standard by which to answer important questions, including how much vitamin D is just enough. As Dr. Manson says, "We already know it's important for bone health to avoid vitamin D deficiency. But once we get to the threshold of 600 to 800

The author
takes 4000 IU of
vitamin D3 daily.

international units (IU) per day, or a blood level of 20 ng/mL, we don't know if getting to higher levels will provide additional benefits or even if the benefits will outweigh the risks."

Vitamin D3 is the only supplement I take regularly. It's simple: If this growing mountain of evidence is wrong and vitamin D3 supplements don't fortify my immune system or decrease the chances I'll eventually be diagnosed with one of many different conditions, then I'll be out about $30 a year. But suppose this growing mountain of evidence is right, and I didn't take a vitamin D3 supplement? That would be a very poor bargain. There is no longer any question that vitamin D plays an important role in maintaining good health and may even prevent an array of disease and conditions. I agree with Creighton University Professor of Medicine Robert Heaney, a specialist in osteoporosis, who said, "Even if two-thirds of these things don't pan out, it's [vitamin D's] still a blockbuster."

3

RUN (OR WALK) FOR YOUR LIFE!

As a physician, perhaps the best advice I can give to my patients is, "Move! Move! And keep moving!" It is indisputable that people who exercise regularly live healthier and longer and lives. In a world in which it is not at all uncommon for a drug to generate revenues of more than a billion dollars a year, it's rare to find something absolutely free that is as good as, or even better for you than, some of the most expensive prescribed medications. Something as simple as a walk in the park can add years to your life. Like the sunshine that creates vitamin D, at least some of the best things in life are readily available at absolutely no cost.

As the *New York Times* explained, "Evidence suggests that our genes evolved to favor exercise. In other words, during prehistoric times, if a person couldn't move quickly and wasn't strong, that person died. Those who were fit survived to reproduce and pass on their 'fitter' genes. Some researchers believe that with our current inactive lifestyle, these genes produce a number of bad effects, which can lead to many chronic illnesses."

Think of it this way: If exercise was a commodity that

Exercise is the best "drug." It has powerful lifesaving effects for people with serious chronic conditions.

could be put into pill, tablet, or liquid form, then bottled and sold, it would instantly become the most commonly prescribed, best-selling, and most beneficial drug in the world. Instead it is absolutely free, and it is as easy as raking leaves in the fall or walking to a nearby java shop for your favorite cup of coffee!

A joint study conducted by Harvard and Stanford Medical Schools and published in the *British Medical Journal* in 2013 analyzed 305 randomized, controlled studies involving 339,274 participants to assess mortality outcomes, comparing the efficacy of exercise and drug interventions with each other or with a control. Researchers found no statistically detectable differences between exercise and drug interventions in the four potentially life-threatening conditions that had been studied: type 2 diabetes, heart failure, repeat stroke, and repeat coronary heart disease. What surprised researchers, according to study director Huseyin Naci, was that "exercise seems to have such powerful life-saving effects for people with serious chronic conditions. It was also surprising to find that so little is known about the potential benefits of physical activity for health in so many other illnesses. What we don't know about the benefits of exercise may be hurting us."

In studies regular physical activity has been shown to reduce the risk of premature death; assist in weight control; and lower the risk of heart disease, type 2 diabetes, stroke, cognitive decline and depression, certain types of cancer, osteoporosis and bone fractures, and even sexual dysfunction.

The most obvious effect of exercise is weight loss and maintenance of that loss. Although exercise without diet control won't allow people to lose significant weight, even those few pounds you can lose by exercising regularly will make a substantial difference in your health. America is facing a large problem—we're in the midst of a burgeoning epidemic of obesity, and a mountain of studies have shown that overweight people get sick and injured far more often than their healthier counterparts and also have shorter life spans. As a hepatologist, in my lectures I note that the dominant liver disease now in America is a condition called nonalcoholic fatty liver disease (NAFLD). It is estimated that forty million Americans have this disorder that is indisputably a consequence of the rise in obesity and type 2 diabetes. Fifteen to twenty percent of patients with NAFLD progress to cirrhosis of the liver and, if they develop complications, become candidates for receiving a liver transplant. It is believed that in the coming decade cirrhosis and complications from NAFLD will be the dominant indication for liver transplantation in the United States.

A research team headed by Dr. Steven Moore of the National Cancer Institute's Nutritional Epidemiology Branch analyzed data collected from more than 650,000 participants in six large studies investigating the association between lifestyle and disease risk. Their results, published in the peer-reviewed online medical journal *PLOS Medicine* in 2013, showed that, compared with sedentary people, those who took a brisk ten-minute daily walk had a life expectancy extended by 1.8 years and that the World Health Organization's recommended 150 minutes of brisk walking weekly could add as much as four and a half years to your life.

More than two decades ago the first report from the surgeon general of the United States on physical activity and health concluded that the benefits of physical activity include "a reduced risk of premature mortality and reduced risk of

Exercising regularly
significantly lowers the
risk of coronary heart disease,
hypertension, and diabetes.

coronary heart disease, hypertension, colon cancer and diabetes mellitus. Regular participation in physical activity also appears to reduce depression and anxiety, improve mood and enhance ability to perform daily tasks throughout the life span." The surgeon general stated flatly, "Higher levels of regular physical activity are associated with lower mortality rates for both older and younger adults, (and) even those who are moderately active on a regular basis have lower mortality rates than those who are least active."

Since then numerous studies have confirmed and even expanded on these conclusions. In 2008, for example, the Department of Health and Human Services issued new guidelines for healthy living based on a meta-analysis of studies done over a long period of time. The thirteen-member panel, which spent more than a year conducting the first comprehensive review of scientific research in more than a decade, concluded that "regular physical activity can cut the risk of heart attacks and stroke by at least 20 percent, reduce chances of an early death and help people avoid high blood pressure, Type 2 diabetes, colon and breast cancer, fractures from age weakening bones, and depression."

The concept that exercise will improve your health and may extend your life is not new; the Greek physician Hippocrates, considered the father of Western medicine, believed, "[i]f we could give every individual the right amount of nourishment and exercise, not too little and not too much, we would have found the safest way to health."

But it has taken a long time to provide conclusive evidence. As far back as 600 BCE Sushruta, a renowned practitioner of the traditional Indian form of medicine called ayurveda, prescribed exercise for his patients, explaining, "it should be taken

Those people who exercise
regularly have a lower risk
of breast and colon cancer
and of depression.

every day," but "only to half extent of his capacity" because it otherwise "may prove fatal." Sushruta recognized the association between exercise and good health, pointing out, "diseases fly from the presence of a person habituated to regular physical exercise." Sushruta advocated moderate exercise and wrote that "[i]t gives the desirable mental qualities of alertness, retentive memory, and keen intelligence."

The basic concept that exercise is vital to good health was well-known in the Middle Ages, when philosopher, physician, and rabbi Moses Maimonides wrote, "As long as one exercises, exerts oneself greatly and does not eat to the point of being full . . . he will not suffer sickness and he will grow in strength."

The more specific suggestion that exercise directly benefits heart health, and thus might increase longevity, appears to have first been made almost two hundred fifty years ago by English physician William Heberden. In 1772 Dr. Heberden identified and described angina as "a disorder of the breast. . . . They who are afflicted with it are seized while they are walking, more especially if it be up hill, and soon after eating with a painful and most disagreeable sensation. . . ." Then he pointed out the odd case of one of his patients, "who set himself the task of sawing wood every day and was nearly cured."

Almost a century later Irish physician William Stokes noted, "the symptoms of debility of the heart are often removable by a regulated course of gymnastics, or by pedestrian exercise." By "pedestrian," he wrote, he meant walking on level ground with the distance and gradient being increased gradually—sort of like working out on a treadmill—while always being wary of excessive fatigue, chest pain, and shortness of breath. But rather than following this suggestion,

throughout the next century most doctors continued to pre-
scribe extended bed rest and limited activity as the best treatment for heart problems.

It wasn't until a landmark study was published in the 1950s
that doctors began to understand the lifesaving relationship
between exercise and heart disease. Just after World War II
the British government noted an increase in the number of
heart attack deaths and wondered about the cause. A scientist
named Jerry Morris designed a study to track the heart attack
rates of people in various civil service occupations. He eventually ended up following more than nine thousand British
civil servants for almost a decade. As he recalled, "The very
first results we got were from the London busmen. And there
was a striking difference in the heart-attack rate. The drivers
of these double-decker buses had substantially more, age for
age, than the conductors." What intrigued Morris was that
these were men from the same social class, working for the
same company under essentially the same conditions. So
he spent hours sitting on buses, watching them do their jobs,
and soon the difference became apparent: "The drivers were
prototypically sedentary, and the conductors were unavoid-
ably active." The conductors, in fact, who suffered roughly
half the number of fatal heart attacks as the drivers, spent
their shifts climbing up and down as many as seven hundred
fifty stairs a day during their shift. While it seems obvious
now, Morris was the first to suggest the direct relationship
between physical activity and heart disease. He subsequently
applied his theory to postmen and found that the men who
delivered the mail by foot or on bicycles had substantially
fewer heart attacks than men their same age and economic
status who sat behind desks in the office. In 1953 the *Lancet*

published the results of his study, which heralded the beginning of the intensive research that was to follow.

In the United States this new concept was brought home to Americans in the mid-1950s when President Dwight Eisenhower suffered a serious heart attack and Mass General cardiologist Dr. Paul Dudley White, one of the founders of the American Heart Association (AHA), warned, "A normal person should exercise seven hours a week."

The medical profession took White's advice and began researching the value of aerobic exercise in preventing heart disease. Among the first studies was the U.S. Railroad Workers Study conducted by the University of Utah Medical School, in which three thousand white, middle-aged railroad workers were followed for twenty years, or until death, beginning in 1957; it was published in the AHA journal *Circulation* in 1988. Researchers concluded that the "data support the notion that physical activity, specifically that done in leisure time, protects against coronary heart disease. Physical activity appears to be directly related to the development of Coronary Heart Disease (CHD), [and] increasing physical activity, particularly of a light-to-moderate intensity, is appropriate to prevent disease and to promote health."

Exercise, for most purposes, is properly defined as physical activity that is planned, structured, and repetitive and has a final or intermediate objective: the improvement of physical fitness. But that definition is actually incomplete, because exercise can include almost all physical activity and also can lead to cognitive improvement as it promotes mental as well as physical fitness. The questions that begged to be answered were how much exercise was enough and what type of exercise was best. When researchers began testing White's conclusion, they discovered that rather than his suggested seven hours, even a moderate amount of exercise could be an effective form of treatment—and not just for heart problems. Other researchers discovered that exercise had a positive effect on a wide range of medical issues, among them depression, anxiety, and even diabetes. While it took an unduly long time, an exercise program has become one of the essential pillars for maintaining good health.

Because heart disease—a broad term used to describe a variety of afflictions affecting the heart—is the leading cause of death for both American men and women, the federal government and the American Heart Association have sponsored numerous studies to try to find the best way to combat it. In 2003, for example, the AHA sponsored a meta-analysis of fifty-two exercise-training trials lasting more than twelve weeks and including 4,700 participants. This summary confirmed previous studies showing that physical activity reduces the incidence of atherosclerotic heart disease—thickening of the arterial blood vessels—overall and helps manage several key factors for heart disease.

A meta-analysis of fifty-one randomized, controlled trials that included 8,440 patients with cardiovascular disease conducted over a period of two and a half years showed that exercising alone decreased mortality by 27 percent. Simply stated, exercise lowered the death rate from heart disease by more than a quarter.

The results of a study published in the *Journal of the American Medical Association* in 2009 proved even more striking: Researchers from the Cardiology Department of New Orleans's Ochsner Clinic Foundation provided one-hour exercise classes three times a week, plus lifestyle advice, for twelve weeks to

Exercise lowers
cardiovascular mortality
by 27 percent.

five hundred cardiac patients, then tracked their progress. Six years later those patients who continued to follow a fitness regime had reduced their chances of dying during that period by 60 percent.

A 2014 Swedish study published in *Circulation* tracked almost forty thousand people who did not have heart failure at the beginning of the study for five years and found that the more active an individual is, the lower his or her risk for heart failure. People who exercised moderately for an hour a day, or vigorously for a half hour daily, cut their risk of heart failure almost by half.

These results did not surprise me. My father was a renowned cardiologist in India who believed there were great benefits to be derived from regular exercise. He encouraged my brother Deepak and I to participate in sports. In fact, when I was nine years old I ran a ten-mile race in Jabalpur, in central India. The students had to be ten years or older to participate. Initially, they wouldn't permit me to run. I asked them, "What if I got my father, a physician, to write a letter to them in which he would say that I was eminently fit to run this race?" They agreed and my father wrote that letter. I was very excited and ran the race with utmost effort. The top ten finishers received prizes—and I finished eleventh. At the award ceremony, I was standing in the stadium and the principal announced that this year they were going to make an exception and award one additional prize to a nine-year-old who had participated in the race and come in eleventh. No wonder I still remember this moment fondly. Throughout my life, I've made physical activity a daily component of my life. As a child, in addition to running, I played cricket, table tennis, and field hockey. For years, I was an avid tennis player, playing four to five times a week and justifying it to my wife by saying I needed to do so for my health!

The benefits of even moderate exercise are not limited to heart disease. One of the proven ways to reduce the risk of being diagnosed with several of the most common forms of cancer is to keep your weight within a safe range. The American Institute for Cancer Research estimates that obesity is among the causes of more than one hundred thousand cases of cancer annually. Here's a startling fact: According to a 2009 report in *Lancet Oncology*, one out of every five women who die from cancer is obese. Keeping your weight within a safe range may reduce your risk of cancer. But apparently the value of exercise in lowering your chances of being diagnosed with certain forms of cancer extend far beyond that. Although the precise mechanism isn't known, Abby Bloch, head of the American Cancer Society's committee on nutrition and physical activity, states flatly, "We now believe physical activity is a primary component of preventing cancer."

As researchers from the National Cancer Institute reported in the *NCI Journal*, "There was consistent evidence from 27 observational studies that physical activity is associated with reduced all-cause, breast cancer-specific, and colon cancer-specific mortality." A 2002 analysis conducted by Cancer Research UK of fifty-one studies concluded that exercising for thirty minutes three or more times weekly could cut the risk of colon cancer by as much as 50 percent, lung cancer by 40 percent, and breast cancer by almost 33 percent and had a favorable impact on the incidence of prostate cancer. An American Cancer Society study confirmed that women who exercised six hours or more weekly cut their risk of breast cancer by 30 percent. Researchers from Kaiser Permanente and

Obesity increases the
risk of developing many cancers,
including breast and colon cancer.

the University of Utah examined the effect of exercise on the risk of developing colon cancer. In their 2003 study published in the *American Journal of Epidemiology*, they found that both men and women who worked out vigorously for more than five hours a week had that same 50 percent reduction in their risk of being diagnosed with colon cancer as seen in the Cancer Research UK 2002 analysis. As Dr. Elizabeth Delasobera, the fellowship program director of sports medicine at Georgetown University Hospital, points out, "43 out of 51 studies demonstrated a decreased risk of colon cancer. In the most physically active participants that risk reduction averaged 40-to-50 percent, up to 70 percent."

As the *NCI Journal* explained, this reduction also is found for breast cancer. A European meta-analysis that included thirty-seven large studies conducted between 1987 and 2013 and that eventually included the records of more than four million women concluded that women of any age who exercise an hour a day or more—including all the walking you normally do—reduce their chances of breast cancer by 12 percent.

In addition to the basic aerobic exercises, weight training and resistance has been shown to have substantial benefits in fighting cancer. A two-decade-long survey of more than eighty-five hundred Swedish men published in 2009 in *Cancer Epidemiology, Biomarkers and Prevention* reported that men who worked out with weights and had high muscle strength reduced their chances of dying from a cancer by more than a third.

Not only can exercise reduce your risk of being diagnosed with cancer, but it can also reduce the risk of recurrence. A study done at Boston's Dana-Farber Cancer Institute and presented at a 2009 conference showed that people with colon cancer reduce the chances of its returning by half when they exercise regularly.

As researchers are discovering, active people are healthier than sedentary people, and the benefits are seen across a wide spectrum of illnesses and conditions. People of all ages who exercise regularly appear to live longer, healthier, and happier lives.

Exercise makes you feel better. In a 1999 Duke University Medical Center experiment sponsored by the NIH, 156 elderly patients diagnosed with serious depression were divided into three groups: one of those groups was treated with medication, a second group was directed to exercise, and the third group took medication and exercised. The medication was the popular antidepressant Zoloft; the exercise component consisted of a thirty-minute walk or jog around a track three times a week. After four months each of the three groups showed roughly the same level of improvement: 60 percent of the patients who exercised only were no longer clinically depressed, compared with 65.5 percent of the patients treated with medication and 68.8 percent of the combination group—although medication did have a positive effect more rapidly than exercise. Duke psychologist James Blumenthal admitted that his research team couldn't explain why exercise alone had such a profound result, but it was impossible not to conclude, "[e]xercise may be just as effective as medication and may be a better alternative for certain patients."

Those results were confirmed in 2007 by investigators at the Mayo Clinic, whose research suggested that moderately intense exercising for a half hour three to five times weekly will "significantly improve depression symptoms," while exercising for less time, ten minutes, can improve your mood for a short term. A 2009 study published in the *Ochsner Foundation Journal* reported that moderate exercise can reduce stress levels by more than half.

While it has long been known that intensive exercise will release "happy" endorphins—the cause of the well-known "runner's high"—that will provide a brief mental boost, there is also evidence that exercise actually builds new brain cells. After researchers at the Salk Institute, in La Jolla, California, demonstrated that exercise causes mice to grow new cells in the area of the brain known to be affected by age-related memory loss, they worked with a Columbia University Medical Center team to conduct a human test. Although it has not yet been possible to show the new cells growing, they proved that in eleven participants aerobic exercise routinely increased blood flow to the area of the brain controlling memory. These tests demonstrated that as each individual became more fit, there was a corresponding increase in blood flow. Arguably the most ambitious study yet done exploring the association between physical activity and executive function— the ability to think in an orderly manner, which is important in mental multitasking, focus, and concentration—in children was conducted by researchers at the University of Illinois at Urbana-Champaign and published in *Pediatrics* in 2014. In this school-year-long study, 220 eight- and nine-year-olds were divided into two groups; one group participated in a two-hour afterschool organized play program as often as they desired, while the other group served as the control group. It should be noted that the control group still got plenty of exercise-play time. In addition to losing body fat, the children in the exercise group showed a substantial improvement in tests of their executive function capabilities. The control group also improved their cognitive scores, as might be expected in growing children, but to a much smaller extent.

Many other studies have shown that exercise can make you smarter. Researchers from the Department of Neurology in Germany's University of Muenster tested the association between exercise and learning ability in twenty-seven healthy adults. Each of the participants was asked to learn a set of vocabulary words directly after a high-impact workout, a low-impact workout, or a rest period. The researchers' conclusion, published in *Neurobiology of Learning and Memory* in 2007, was that "vocabulary learning was 20 percent faster after intense physical exercise as compared to the other two conditions . . . [and] [r]egular physical exercise improves cognitive functions and lowers the risk for age-related cognitive decline."

Several studies have shown that these cognitive benefits are not restricted to young people. Another University of Illinois at Urbana-Champaign study, this one done in conjunction with Israel's Bar-Ilan University and published in *Nature* in 1999, divided one hundred twenty previously sedentary adults from ages sixty to seventy-five into two groups, one guided through a six-month program of aerobic (walking) exercises, the other given anaerobic (stretching and toning) exercises, and found "those who received aerobic training showed substantial improvements in performance on tasks requiring executive control compared with anaerobically trained subjects."

In 2009 researchers at Medical University of South Carolina Children's Hospital designed a study in which one hundred five students at a Charleston elementary school who had been exercising forty minutes a week instead exercised forty

Vocabulary learning is significantly faster after intense physical exercise. It can make us smarter!

minutes daily, with age-appropriate academic content available on TV screens as they worked out. At the end of the year the Pediatric Academic Societies concluded that test scores had increased 13 percent compared with the previous year.

A 2013 study conducted by the Department of Psychology and Brain Health Research Centre at New Zealand's University of Otago and published in *Psychonomic Bulletin & Review* concluded, "Data to date from studies of aging provide strong evidence of exercise-linked benefits related to task switching, selective attention, inhibition of prepotent responses, and working memory capacity."

Exercise doesn't just make it easier to perform mental tasks, it also appears to help seniors retain information. An analysis of three large international studies published in the *Archives of Internal Medicine* in 2009 reported, "Risk of impaired performance on the six-item Cognitive Impairment Test . . . of about 3,900 people 55 and older was cut nearly in half among people with moderate or high levels of physical activity."

While the precise reasons for many of the physiological benefits of exercise haven't been established, the irrefutable fact is that it can make a big difference in preventing or moderating many diseases or conditions. For example, exercise can reduce the risk of your being diagnosed with type 2 diabetes, a serious disease that is rapidly becoming commonplace, by a significant number. According to the Centers for Disease Control, "Research studies have found that moderate weight loss and exercise can prevent or delay type 2 diabetes among adults at high-risk of diabetes." Beyond showing that exercise fights heart disease, that 2003 American Heart Association study concluded that losing an average of 8.8 pounds and walking six miles a week, "reduced the onset of Type 2 diabetes in individuals at high risk for this disease by 58 percent compared with the usual care." A 2007 meta-analysis by the Polish Academy of Physical Education looked at studies published in the previous three years and confirmed a "[r]isk reduction of 49 percent for cardiovascular and heart disease, 35 percent for diabetes," and a strong impact in reducing the risk of being diagnosed with either breast or colorectal cancer.

One of the largest studies investigated the ability of muscle-strengthening exercises to prevent type 2 diabetes. A team of researchers from several major institutions, including the Harvard School of Public Health and Brigham and Women's Hospital in Boston, examined data from 99,316 middle-aged and elderly women who were followed for a minimum of eight years in the Nurses' Health Study and Follow-Up. The results, published in *PLOS* online in 2014, found that "women who did more than 150 min/week of these types of exercise (weight training, yoga, aerobics and similar exercises) had 40% lower risk of developing diabetes as women who did not exercise in this way at all. Muscle-strengthening and muscle-conditioning exercise were both independently associated with reduced diabetes risk, and women who engaged in at least 150 minutes weekly of aerobic MVPA and at least 60 minutes weekly of muscle-strengthening exercise were a third as likely to develop diabetes as inactive women."

There can be no doubt that regular exercise should be part of everyone's life. While most children get sufficient exercise by playing, as we get older and our lives become filled with work and other responsibilities, we struggle to find the time to exercise. As a result we become less active at the time we probably need it most. The benefits of exercise are cumulative; fit people live longer. But as we age, exercise also makes a significant difference in our ability to enjoy life. In the Lifestyle Interventions and Independence for Elders (LIFE) Study, researchers from eight universities and research centers across the nation recruited 1,635 men and women between the ages of seventy and eighty-nine with very limited mobility. These participants, who at the start of the trial were sedentary and infirm, people who might accurately be described as frail, were assigned to either an exercise or an education group. The exercise group was asked to walk about two and a half hours a week and complete thirty minutes of light weight training. The experiment continued for an average of two and a half years. At the end of that time, as reported in *JAMA* in 2014, those people who exercised regularly were about 18 percent less likely to have had a single episode of physical disability and about 28 percent less likely to have developed a persistent or permanent disability. As the lead author of the study, Dr. Marco Pahor, the director of the Institute on Aging at the University of Florida in Gainesville, explained, "we have directly shown that exercise can effectively lessen or prevent the development of physical disability in a population of extremely vulnerable elderly people[;] . . . these exercises have an important public health impact."

The 2009 Jerusalem Longitudinal Cohort Study provided similar results, concluding that even for elderly people moderate exercise—more than four hours weekly—decreased mortality and improved function. This eighteen-year-long study followed almost two thousand people born prior to 1921 and found that for seventy-year-olds who engaged in four hours of exercise weekly, mortality decreased over an eight-year period by 12 percent, by almost 15 percent for seventy-eight-year-olds, and by about 20 percent for those eight-five or older. Equally important, at all ages there was a measureable difference in the ability to continue daily activities. As one investigator emphasized, "Not only was the effect of this benefit similar regardless of advancing age but the magnitude of the difference between physically active and sedentary (less than four hours of exercise weekly) participants actually increased with advancing age."

An analysis of data from 13,500 participants in the Nurses' Health Study, published in *Archives of Internal Medicine*, reported similar results in 2009: "[T]he likelihood of successful survival [living past seventy, in general good physical and mental health] was nearly doubled for those who had been in the highest quintile [20 percent] of overall physical activity 10 to 15 years earlier than for the most sedentary participants."

There is simply no doubt that every one of us should be physically active as much and as often as possible. It isn't hard to incorporate more activity in your daily life without it becoming burdensome. I have heard best-selling author Dr. Michael Roizen, chief wellness officer of the renowned Cleveland Clinic, tell other physicians, "the single best thing you can do for your patients is urge them to buy a pedometer." This is a device that enables people to count the steps they take. Pedometers now perform a variety of tasks, from counting the number of steps taken to counting calories burned. The Nike FuelBand and the Fitbit are among the most popular brands. What these devices do, essentially, is allow you to set a measureable daily standard and monitor it easily, competing with yourself or others to match it or do more. Most importantly, they serve to remind you to take that extra step. Exercise is not limited to the gym: in a building you can choose to walk up stairs rather than taking an elevator or escalator; you can walk to the nearby store rather than taking a short drive; in a parking lot you can find a spot far away from your destination and walk to get there—I always find it ironic that people drive to a gym then try to park as close as possible to the front door. The one thing I must tell you is that exercise is *not* how many times you can walk back and forth to the refrigerator or the wine cellar!

There is no secret formula that equates the type of exercise you choose and the length of time you do it to a specific result. Each person gets individual benefits based on his or her own physical situation. But the best news is that exercise is something you can try at home. Dr. Qi Sun of the Harvard School of Public Health, and the lead author of the Nurses' Health Study findings about exercise, published in *JAMA* in 2010, said that for women, "In terms of magnitude, walking and other moderate activities were almost equivalent to the benefit gained from more vigorous physical activity."

Probably the simplest form of exercise is walking—and fortunately it also happens to among the most beneficial. Walking is so easy even a baby can do it—but it does provide substantial benefits. The Nurses' Health Study tracked 72,000 women for two decades and reported that walking briskly for three hours a week, a half hour a day, can reduce a woman's risk of a heart attack by as much as 40 percent. Similarly, the Harvard Alumni Health Study, published in *JAMA* in 1995, followed 11,000 male alumni for sixteen years and determined that walking one hour five days a week might cut the risk of having a stroke by half. Walking also builds bone strength, which is extremely important as we age; a 2014 Harvard Medical School and Brigham and Women's Hospital study published in the *American Journal of Public Health* analyzed twenty-four years of data from about 36,000 participants in the Health Professionals Follow-Up Study and reported that men over fifty years old who walked more than four hours a week reduced their risk of fracturing a hip by 43 percent over men who walked less than four hours—and those who self-reported walking at a brisk pace reduced their risk by 63 percent.

There has been a lot of speculation about the health benefits of walking compared with high-impact exercises like running, biking, and swimming. Consider walking a baseline exercise: it is an exercise activity that people of all ages can do and enjoy. An interesting study directed by Paul T. Williams, a scientist at Lawrence Berkeley National Laboratory, Life Science Division, in Berkeley, California, and published in 2013 in the AHA magazine *Arteriosclerosis, Thrombosis and Vascular Biology,* compared results from 33,060 runners in the National Runners' Health Study and 15,045 walkers in the National Walkers' Health Study. As Williams explained, "Walking and running provide an ideal test of the health benefits of moderate-intensity walking and vigorous-intensity running because they involve the same muscle groups and the same activities performed at different intensities." Unlike previous studies, this one compared results based on distance covered, not the time it took. So while walkers may take twice as long as runners to cover a similar distance, it appears the benefits they get are equal and in some areas even better. The six-year-long study found that when runners and walkers expended the same amount of energy they saw similar reductions in their risk for high blood pressure, high cholesterol, diabetes, and possibly coronary heart disease. For example, walking reduced coronary heart disease

Walking, perhaps the simplest form of exercise, is proven to have a multitude of health benefits.

9.3 percent, while running a similar distance reduced the risk by 4.5 percent.

For those people who can run, it provides significant health benefits in addition to the mental boost. In a 2014 study published in the *Journal of American Cardiology,* researchers from several universities and institutions analyzed the health records of 55,137 healthy men and women from eighteen to one hundred years old and discovered that in the fifteen years before the study began the risk of runners dying from any cause was 30 percent lower than for nonrunners, while the risk of dying from a heart-related problem was lower for runners by 45 percent. Runners lived about three years longer than nonrunners, and even overweight smokers who ran were less likely to die prematurely. Equally interesting was the fact that the benefits were roughly equal no matter how long you ran, as people who reported running only a few minutes got generally the same benefits as those people who ran for a considerably longer period of time.

Aerobic exercises are especially good for your heart, but they do little to increase your upper-body strength. Working with weights or resistance may also provide cardiac benefits, and it is extremely important in building and maintaining bone and muscle strength and flexibility. Adults can lose as much as 8 percent of their muscle mass a decade, which leads directly to a loss of mobility and strength and can result in fractured and broken bones. In a 2014 story published in the Harvard Medical School's publication *HEARTbeat Archive,* "strength training (with free weights, weight machines, or resistance bands) can help build and maintain muscle mass and strength. What many of us don't know is that strong muscles lead to strong bones. And strong bones can help minimize the risk of fracture due to osteoporosis.

"Numerous studies have shown that strength training can play a role in slowing bone loss, and several show it can even build bone. This is tremendously useful to help offset age-related decline in bone mass. . . . What's more, resistance workouts—particularly those that include moves emphasizing power and balance—enhance strength and stability. That can boost confidence, encourage you to stay active, and reduce fractures by cutting down on falls."

The American Heart Association admits that before 1990 resistance training was not part of its guidelines for training or rehabilitation; it has since been recognized as a significant component of a comprehensive fitness program for healthy adults of all ages. The AHA currently advises that "[m]ild-to-moderate resistance training can provide an effective method for improving muscular strength and endurance, preventing and managing a variety of chronic medical conditions, modifying coronary risk factors, and enhancing psychosocial well-being."

While aerobic exercises tend to reduce the risk of certain illnesses and diseases, by building bone strength weight-bearing exercises and resistance training help rebuild or maintain the skeletal system and prevent loss of mobility and specific diseases like arthritis and osteoporosis. According to a 2007 statement from the Centers for Disease Control, strength training—lifting weights and using resistance—provided significant relief from the symptoms of arthritis by decreasing pain 43 percent, "increased muscle strength and general physical performance, improved the clinical signs and symptoms of the disease and decreased disability." This proves that "[t]he effectiveness of strength training to ease the pain of osteoporosis was just as potent, if not more potent, than medications." This same meta-analysis demonstrated that strength training also increases bone density, has a "profound impact on helping older adults manage diabetes[,] . . . provides similar improvements in depression as anti-depression medications," and reduces heart disease.

In addition, several reliable studies have shown that strength-training programs may also help participants improve their balance, which will reduce the risk of falls, which lead too often to fractures—especially in the elderly. The Division of Arthritis and Rheumatic Diseases at Oregon Health and Sciences University reports, "Exercise in the form of short, repetitive mechanical loading leads to the greatest gains in bone strength."

The NIH-sponsored National Institute of Arthritis and Musculoskeletal Diseases' Bone Estrogen and Strength Tests were conducted by the Departments of Physiology and Nutritional Sciences at the University of Arizona between 1995 and 2001. For this study 266 postmenopausal women averaging fifty-six years old were randomly assigned to an exercise group or a control group. While all the women received a calcium supplement, the exercise group met three times weekly for a year to perform supervised weight-bearing and weight-lifting exercises. At the end of that year researchers reported, "Weight bearing and resistance exercises over a one-year period, combined with calcium supplementation, significantly improved bone mineral density at skeletal sites at risk for osteoporotic fractures in postmenopausal women." In fact, rather than losing bone mineral density, a cause of osteoporosis, they actually improved it by 1 to 2 percent.

Exercise has proven to be so important that some doctors have literally begun prescribing exercise for their patients. Dr. Eddie Phillips, a physician working at the Joslin Diabetes Center and an assistant professor of physical medicine and rehabilitation at Harvard Medical School, asks his patients which exercise they most enjoy, then writes the prescription for them: twenty minutes, three times weekly. There is evidence that this somewhat whimsical approach works: The *Scandinavian Journal of Medicine & Science in Sports* reported that 6,300 patients who had been leading a sedentary lifestyle or who were suffering from a condition that would benefit from exercise, like high cholesterol or diabetes, were given prescriptions by their doctors to exercise. These activities included walking, organized aerobics, or weight lifting. At the end of a year more than half of these patients reported being more active than they had been at the beginning of the study. A third of them reported that they were currently exercising regularly, and almost 15 percent who initially had described themselves as inactive reported they were exercising regularly.

While the concept of exercising has caught hold in America and led to an explosion in the number of fitness clubs and individuals participating in a range of activities from aerobics to zumba, this country is still facing an epidemic of obesity. According to a 2013 article published in *BMJ*, an astonishing 80 percent of Americans eighteen and older failed to meet the recommended levels of aerobic and muscle-strengthening physical activities.

So what exercises should you be doing, and how often and how long should you be doing them for? It's probable that few people are going to suddenly make the decision that they need to begin exercising then find a way to carve hours out of their

An exercise prescription:
Walk or swim for thirty minutes
three times a week.
Number of refills: infinite!

schedule and change their entire lifestyle. It rarely happens that way. The best way to begin may be to substitute the word "activity" for "exercise": just start moving more than you normally do in your everyday life.

As the ancient Chinese philosopher Lao-tzu once said, "A journey of a thousand miles begins with a single step." Don't set grand goals, start slowly, and ease into it. Something is much better than nothing. The best advice for normally sedentary people is to incorporate these changes into their life slowly, don't try to do too much too fast. The good news is that they'll actually begin seeing benefits by adding as little as ten minutes a day of moderately intensive exercise—without any risk. As New York City personal trainer and yoga instructor Laura Stevens points out to her clients, "You can walk ten minutes a day now or end up sitting in your doctor's office later."

How much exercise is the right amount? A 2008 Health and Human Services report set the minimum to achieve good health for adults at two and a half hours weekly of moderate aerobic activity—or half of that if you're doing a vigorous exercise like jogging, playing soccer, bicycling, or swimming. The American Heart Association recommends one hundred fifty minutes of moderate activity or seventy-five minutes of vigorous activity weekly to derive benefits. That means if you walk fast, swim, garden, or even go ballroom dancing for twenty minutes a day you'll meet those minimum guidelines. And the fact is that no matter what is recommended, the more you work out, the better it is for you.

While generally tests indicate strength training is most beneficial when done three times a week for about a half hour, there is some research that indicates "a single set of 12 repetitions with the proper weight can build muscle just as efficiently as three sets of the same exercise." The key to that, according to Dr. Edward Laskowski, the codirector of the Mayo Clinic's Sports Medicine Center, is that "[a]t the proper weight, you should be just barely able to finish the 12th repetition."

Some studies have shown that turning your workouts into social events with your friends and family increases the likelihood that you will exercise regularly. People who regularly work out with someone else tend to be more diligent about showing up and also seem to work out a bit longer and enjoy it more. Personally, in addition to playing golf as often as possible, I work out with my friends three or four times a week. I do it because I enjoy the company of my friends, but knowing they are waiting for me makes it possible for me to meet them at 6:30 in the morning, even on those mornings when I might like to skip it—just this one time. And honestly, there isn't a time after I've finished my workout that I wasn't pleased that I had shown up and gone through it.

Obviously, I'm not alone. Fitness has become a huge industry. By 2012 there were about 30,500 health clubs in America with more than fifty million members. But no one has to join a health club to exercise. There are many ways to integrate exercise into your normal activities. For example:

- If you are taking an elevator to the tenth floor, get off on the seventh or eighth and walk up two or three flights.
- If you have to travel a short distance, don't drive. Walk or bike to the destination.
- Park your car as far as possible from the entrance to the shopping mall or gym.

- Take your dog for a walk.
- Consider getting a treadmill desk so that while you're working you can be walking on the treadmill at a slow speed.
- Wear a pedometer and track the number of steps you take each day. For those of us who like feedback, this can be enormously helpful.
- Use a stationary bicycle or treadmill while watching TV.
- Get an exercise buddy. That person could be thousands of miles away, but you exchange e-mails or text each other about how you are going to go exercise and how you triumphantly did so!

While the existing evidence is already extremely strong, the importance of exercise in maintaining good health is a relatively new field of research. There have been an abundance of studies demonstrating the association, but there are more exciting discoveries being made and published every day. So let me paraphrase an old saying: Rather than exercising good sense, it makes good sense for you to exercise.

4
Nuts to You!

A hundred years ago famed agricultural scientist Luther Burbank wrote, "The chemical analysis of their [nuts'] constituents shows that they are in the main highly concentrated foods, having little waste aside from their shells. They contain all the important constituents of diet—proteins, fats and carbohydrates—and are thus in themselves capable of sustaining life. They do not contain the various elements in proper proportion, however, to make them suitable for an exclusive diet."

The first nut was cracked open millions of years ago, and since that time the various varieties of nuts have been an important staple of the human diet. Israeli archeologists have found seven types of nuts and the stones needed to break them open that had been buried almost eight hundred thousand years ago. Remains of pecans eaten in 6100 BC have been found in Texas. In 2838 BC Chinese scholars listed the hazelnut as one of the five sacred foods that the gods had bestowed upon human beings. The Babylonian king Nebuchadnezzar decreed that pistachio trees should be planted in the legendary hanging gardens. Almonds are mentioned in the Old Testa-

Nuts are a powerhouse
of nutrition and provide a wide
array of health benefits.

ment. Over three thousand years ago the Incas included peanuts in burial ceremonies so the deceased would have food on
the journey to the beyond. The Greeks and Romans considered nuts food for the gods, and pine nuts to be an aphrodisiac.
Nuts were among the first delicacies brought to the New
World. George Washington planted pecan trees given to him
by Thomas Jefferson at Mount Vernon. Peanuts first came to
America from Africa on slave ships and helped sustain both
Union and Confederate soldiers throughout the Civil War.

Nuts have played an important role in the survival of mankind almost throughout the history of life on earth. But it is
only recently that scientists have begun to appreciate all the
health benefits packed so snugly into that small powerhouse of
nutrition. At a dinner party not too long ago, I was extolling
the virtues of nuts. A friend was listening intently and re-
minded me that good things come in small packages. It turns
out that nuts are like miniature health food stores; as Burbank
surmised, in their chemical makeup nuts have proteins, fats,
fiber, natural-plant omega-3 polyunsaturated fats, phytonutri-
ents, antioxidants like vitamins B and E, selenium, and magnesium.

Throughout history civilizations knew that nuts tasted
good and could be used for a variety of purposes such as a
paste, bowls, and currency. Only recently though has there
been light shed on the multitude of health benefits when nuts
are consumed on a regular basis. In fact, for a long time in
America nuts were believed to be bad for you because they
contained high levels of fat. But as researchers have proved,
the types of fats found in nuts are actually very good for you.

Making nuts a part of your diet has been linked to an array
of health benefits, including lowering the risk of developing

heart disease as well as being diagnosed with several types of cancers. Nuts also lower cholesterol and blood pressure, improve men's reproductive health and even—contrary to the common belief—help individuals lose rather than gain weight.

By definition tree nuts are the seeds of a fruit surrounded by a hard shell—and that shell has to be broken to get to the edible seed. The exceptions to that are the peanut, arguably the most popular of all nuts, which is actually a legume, a close relative to peas and beans, and the largest known seed, the coconut, which technically is a drupe, a fleshy fruit like a peach that surrounds the seed. Because nuts are seeds and the entire source of energy for the new plants, it makes perfect sense that they would be rich in nutrients.

Nuts grow in temperate climates around the world, and different types tend to favor certain places. Pecans, for example, grow mostly in the American Southwest, while about 90 percent of all pistachios are grown in Turkey and Iran. There are conflicting estimates of how many different types of true nuts exist, ranging from as low as fifty to more than one thousand varieties of pecan trees. Nuts do grow on trees: Brazil nut trees can be more than one hundred fifty feet tall and eight feet in diameter and can live more than five hundred years; pecan trees have been known to survive one thousand years, and while peanuts flower above ground, the nuts actually grow in the soil.

Because many of us have the feeling that if something really tastes good it's probably bad for us, the fact that a variety of nuts really should be part of every healthy diet has come as a welcome and pleasant surprise. It is only recently that researchers began taking a good hard look at the nutritional value of nuts. Doctors first became aware of the potential nutritional value of nuts as recently as 1992 with the publication of the Adventist Health Study in the *Archives of Internal Medicine*. The authors of that study concluded, "nut consumption reduces the risk of both fatal and nonfatal coronary heart disease." Researchers at California's Loma Linda University collected health data from 31,208 non-Hispanic white California Seventh-Day Adventists for twelve years. This study was conducted by Loma Linda researchers with the cooperation of the church. At the beginning of the study researchers compiled extensive dietary information from participants in addition to other already known coronary risk factors—smoking, for example—enabling them to break down the results into groups with similar lifestyles and medical conditions. Participants were given different kinds of nuts to eat: slightly less than a third ate peanuts, 29 percent ate almonds, 16 percent walnuts, and 23 percent were given other varieties.

The results were both surprising and conclusive: "Our data strongly suggest that the frequent consumption of nuts may protect against risk of coronary heart disease. . . . Subjects who consumed nuts . . . more than four times a week . . . experienced substantially fewer definite coronary risk factors. . . . These findings were seen in almost all 16 subgroups of the population," which included men and women of all ages and weights as well as people who exercised frequently or rarely. Participants who ate nuts one to four times a week reduced their risk of suffering a fatal heart attack by 27 percent compared with people who ate nuts less than once a week and reduced their risk of having a nonfatal heart attack by 26 percent. But the protective value of nuts was even more pronounced in people who ate nuts five or more times weekly. They reduced their chances of suffering a fatal heart attack by 48 percent and a nonfatal heart attack by more than half. Those people whose daily diet included nuts had an astonishing 60 percent fewer heart attacks than people who ate them less than once a month. There seemed to be no measureable differences in the results based on the type of nuts that were eaten.

The publication of this study focused new attention on nuts, which had long been considered a snack food best eaten in moderation as eating too many nuts was believed to cause weight gain. Nuts for heart health? That sounded, well, nuts! But when other studies produced similar results people began paying heed. One of the singular studies was the Iowa Women's Health Study, published in the *New England Journal of Medicine* in 1996, which reported that postmenopausal women who ate nuts at least four times weekly reduced their chances of dying from a heart attack by 40 percent and, just as in the Adventist study, people who ate nuts five or more times weekly reduced their risk by more than 50 percent.

Any lingering doubt that nuts play a very important role in heart health was dispelled in 1998 with the release of the Nurses' Health Study in the *British Medical Journal*. The Nurses' Health Study is the largest epidemiological study conducted to assess long-term health of women. Beginning in 1976, it included 121,700 registered nurses, although the dietary component didn't begin until 1980. The cohort study of the value of eating nuts followed 86,016 women for eighteen years and found that "[f]requent nut consumption was associated with a reduced risk of both fatal coronary heart disease and non-fatal myocardial infarction."

That same year the Physicians' Health Study, in which 22,000 male physicians were followed for eleven years, found

Consuming nuts lowers the
risk of coronary artery disease.

that "as nut consumption increased, the risk of total cardiac death and sudden death decreased." At the 1998 American Heart Association Conference, researchers from Harvard reported, "These data in U.S. physicians suggest that nut consumption is associated with a reduced risk of total and sudden cardiac death."

The cumulative evidence was so strong that in 2003 the FDA allowed manufacturers to include on packages of nuts the claim, "Scientific evidence suggests but does not prove that eating 1.5 oz per day (about a handful) of most nuts as part of a diet low in saturated fat and cholesterol may reduce the risk of heart disease."

Since then there have been several studies trying to determine exactly why nuts have this protective value. A 2008 Spanish study concluded that nuts might actually be more beneficial to heart patients than olive oil, which has long been valued for its benefits. The twelve hundred participants in the PREDIMED (Prevención con Dieta Mediterránea) study, published in the *Archives of Internal Medicine*, included 751 men and women with metabolic syndrome, a cluster of conditions including excess body fat around the waist, increased blood pressure, a high blood sugar level, and high cholesterol levels. When these conditions occur concurrently, the risk of heart disease, stroke, and type 2 diabetes increases. In the United States, 44 percent of the population over fifty has metabolic syndrome. The study participants were divided into three groups: a group that was given advice about how to reduce fats in their diet, a second group that followed the Mediterranean diet—meaning they increased consumption of fish, fruits, and vegetables; substituted white meat for red meat; included aromatic herbs; and did their cooking in four or more tablespoons of olive oil—and a third group that followed the same diet but also ate nuts regularly.

In the one-year follow-up the group supplementing the Mediterranean diet with peanuts showed a significant 13.7 percent reduction in the prevalance of metabolic syndrome. The group taking additional olive oil saw its risk reduced by 6.7 percent. And the control group had only a 2 percent decrease. The researchers concluded that "a non–energy-restricted traditional MedDiet [Mediterranean diet] enriched with nuts, which is high in fat, high in unsaturated fat, and palatable, is a useful tool in managing the MetS [metabolic syndrome]."

Scientists strongly suspect that at least one reason nuts offer protection against heart disease is that most nuts are packed with protein and unsaturated fats known to lower dangerous LDL cholesterol. After vegetable oils, nuts are richest among all plant foods in fat, ranging from 46 percent fat found in cashews and pistachios to 76 percent in macadamia nuts—more than half of them beneficial fats. Researchers at Penn State conducted a small study of the ability of pistachio nuts to lower bad cholesterol by adding nuts to the subjects' diet regimen and reported that two servings a day added to a low-fat diet reduced cholesterol levels by 12 percent.

A study published in 2010 in the *Archives of Internal Medicine* collected data from twenty-five studies in which 583 people were divided into two groups; one group ate nuts while a control group abstained. The group eating nuts had a 7.4 percent reduction in LDL cholesterol and a similar reduction in the ratio of good-to-bad cholesterol.

Walnuts and almonds in particular have both been found to help reduce cholesterol. A small clinical trial held at the

University of Toronto in 2002 and published in *Circulation* monitored twenty-seven men and women with high cholesterol for three months. Those participants who ate a handful of almonds daily lowered their LDL cholesterol by 4.4 percent—and those people who ate two handfuls saw their LDL levels drop by 9.4 percent. The director of the trial, Dr. David Jenkins, concluded, "Almonds used as snacks in the diets of hyperlipidemic subjects significantly reduce coronary heart disease risk factors, probably in part because of the nonfat (protein and fiber) and monounsaturated fatty acid components of the nut. . . . The combination of monounsaturates with some polyunsaturates in nuts is an ideal combination of fats, all of which may have a beneficial effect on blood cholesterol."

Another nut study conducted by Dr. Jenkins, and published in the *American Journal of Clinical Nutrition* in 2005, tested almonds and other foods against cholesterol-lowering statins. Thirty-four adults with unhealthy high LDL were tested over three one-month periods, and Dr. Jenkins found that a healthy diet including almonds reduced dangerous cholesterol by about 30 percent, only just slightly less than the statins and without any of the potential side effects.

While studies have proved that eating nuts is heart smart and can effectively reduce the risk of heart disease anywhere from 25 percent to 50 percent, there is also evidence that nuts can provide other health benefits. For example, another arm of the Nurses' Health Study investigated the relationship between eating nuts and type 2 diabetes. In results published in *JAMA* in 2002, researchers concluded that eating nuts or peanut butter "suggested potential benefits of higher nut and peanut butter consumption in lowering risk of Type 2 diabe-

Eating nuts can
lower LDL cholesterol
(the "bad" cholesterol).

tes in women." In fact, women who ate a full helping of nuts five or more times a week reduced their risk of being diagnosed with type 2 diabetes by 27 percent, and even those women who enjoyed nuts only once a week saw a modest 8 percent reduction compared with women who did not eat nuts.

The 2008 Shanghai Women's Health Study, as reported in the *American Journal of Clinical Nutrition,* followed 64,000 women with no history of type 2 diabetes for almost five years and concluded, "Our study agrees with the Nurses' Health Study II, which found that consumption of both peanuts and peanut butter was protective against the development of Type 2 diabetes."

Somewhat surprisingly, while the Physicians' Health Study published in the *European Journal of Clinical Nutrition* in 2010 clearly showed that eating nuts reduced the risk of heart disease for men, it did not associate eating nuts with any decrease in the risk of diabetes.

A small but interesting 2014 Spanish study published in *Diabetes Care* divided fifty-four prediabetic adults into two groups. Prediabetic people have high blood sugar and if they do nothing about it as many as a third will develop type 2 diabetes within five years. One group was given about two ounces of pistachio nuts daily, while the control group was given additional olive oil and other fats. After four months the fasting blood sugar levels, insulin, and hormonal markers of insulin resistance had decreased in the pistachio group while they had risen in the control group. According to Dr. Emilio Ros, director of the Lipid Clinic at Hospital Clinic in Barcelona, "Although pistachios were examined in this work, I believe that any beneficial effects on glucose metabolism are shared by all nuts, as they have a general composition with lots of bioactive compounds liable to beneficially affect biological pathways leading to insulin resistance and diabetes."

In several studies nuts also appear to reduce the risk of being diagnosed with certain types of cancer. The Nurses' Health Study associated nuts with a greatly reduced risk of pancreatic cancer. A Harvard Medical School and Brigham and Woman's Hospital study of that data, which followed more than seventy-five thousand women and was published in the *British Journal of Cancer* in 2013, found that "women who consumed a 1 oz serving size of nuts two or more times per week experienced a significantly lower risk of pancreatic cancer when compared with those who largely abstained from nuts." The inverse association persisted within strata defined by body mass index (BMI), physical activity, smoking, and estimated intake of red meats, fruits, and vegetables.

Many scientists have long been intrigued by the possibility that high levels of selenium can reduce chances of developing advanced prostate cancer. At the 2013 meeting of the American Association of Cancer Research, investigators from Maastricht University in the Netherlands presented preliminary data from a study of sixty thousand men that showed those people with a high level of selenium reduce their risk of developing that dangerous cancer by more than 60 percent. Brazil nuts, especially, are high in selenium.

Researchers in Taiwan investigated the link between nuts and colon cancer. The results of their ten-year study of twenty-four thousand men and women, published in the *World Journal of Gastroenterology*, found that women who ate peanuts two or more times weekly reduced their risk of developing colon

Nut consumption can significantly lower the risk of the deadly pancreatic cancer.

cancer by 58 percent, while men saw a significantly lower but still impressive 27 percent reduction in risk.

Results like these have intrigued scientists who have begun investigating possible associations between nuts and cancers. In animal tests, for example, they have found that pistachios may provide at least some protection against lung cancer.

In fact, taken overall there seems to be good evidence that eating nuts will help you live longer. A 2013 report from the Dana-Farber Cancer Institute, in conjunction with Brigham and Women's Hospital and the Harvard School of Public Health and published in the *New England Journal of Medicine,* concluded that people who regularly enjoyed a handful of nuts were 20 percent less likely to die from any cause over a thirty-year period than those who didn't consume nuts. This very large study, supported by the NIH and the nut industry, mined the data on 76,464 women collected over thirty years by the Nurses' Health Study and 42,498 men followed for twenty-four years in the Health Professionals Follow-Up Study. The first author of the report, Ying Bao of Brigham and Women's Hospital, explained, "In all these analyses, the more nuts people ate the less likely they were to die over the 30-year follow-up period." Compared with people who didn't eat nuts at all, those who ate nuts less than once a week still saw a 7 percent reduction in mortality while participants who ate nuts every day reduced their death rate by 20 percent. While there were significant reductions in deaths from cancer, heart disease, and respiratory diseases, the death rate was lower in just about every category. It didn't seem to matter which type of nut was eaten; people who ate nuts lived longer, and the

*2013 Harvard Medical
School study: Over a
thirty-year period,
people who regularly ate a
handful of nuts were 20 percent
less likely to die compared
to those who didn't.*

more nuts they ate the longer they lived. As Bao admitted, no one yet knows why this is true: "The exact biological mechanisms are unclear at this point."

The authors of an early study reached a similar conclusion. The Seventh-Day Adventist study done by Loma Linda University, following up its earlier coronary study, followed 34,192 men and women for twelve years. Published in the *Archives of Internal Medicine* in 2001, the authors concluded that eating nuts on a regular basis resulted in a gain of one and half to two and half years in life expectancy.

While researchers have yet to pinpoint the specific elements in nuts that contribute to their health benefits, unquestionably the most unexpected discovery appears to be that eating nuts may help people either lose weight or maintain their current weight. It has long been accepted that if you eat too many nuts you gain weight. Each cashew, for example, contains about eight or nine calories. An almond has seven calories, and a pistachio has three calories. In fact, many people are so concerned about the number of calories in nuts and the potential weight gain that they don't eat nuts regularly. The really goods news is many studies now indicate that little weight gain comes from eating nuts. A 2013 Spanish meta-analysis of thirty-one studies found that the majority of participants in those studies gained little or no weight and that "nuts—as part of a healthy, balanced diet—can help to stabilize insulin and suppress hunger." Those participants who replaced foods in their diets with nuts lost an average of 1.4 pounds and half an inch from their waist. The report, published in *American Journal of Clinical Nutrition,* concluded, "Although the magnitude of these effects was modest, the results allay the fear that nut consumption may promote obesity."

In fact, another Spanish study, this one conducted by the Department of Preventive Medicine and Public Health at the University of Navarra and published in *Obesity* in 2007, tracked 8,865 participants for twenty-eight months. The investigators reported that participants who ate nuts twice or more weekly reduced their chances of gaining weight by 31 percent compared with those people who abstained, and among those people who did gain weight participants who ate nuts at least two times a week gained about half the amount of those people who never ate nuts.

Purdue professor of foods and nutrition Richard Mattes, PhD, has been investigating the nutritional value of nuts for more than a decade. His 2003 study, "Peanut Consumption Improves Indices of Cardiovascular Risk Disease," published in the *Journal of the American College of Nutrition*, involved fifteen healthy adults who participated in a three-phase, thirty-week trial. In the first trial participants replaced five hundred daily calories from dietary fat with five hundred calories of peanuts. In the second trial participants didn't change their regular diet but added five hundred calories of peanuts. In the third trial participants incorporated peanuts into their diet in any way that was comfortable. All three groups saw a significant reduction—as much as 24 percent—in their triglyceride level, a key risk factor for heart disease, but equally fascinating, according to Professor Mattes, "We saw no significant change in body weight, despite adding 500 calories of peanuts a day for eight weeks."

A decade later Mattes published the results of a similar study in the *European Journal of Clinical Nutrition*. In this study 137 adults at risk for type 2 diabetes were divided into five groups, ranging from one group that ate no nuts and seeds to groups that ate 1.5 ounces of almonds every day for a month. Among other benefits, the author confirmed, "Almonds, consumed as snacks, also reduced hunger and desire to eat during the acute-feeding session. . . . Acute and longer-term almond ingestion helps regulate body weight. . . ."

These results don't seem logical: How can nuts be packed with fat yet people who eat them—and sometimes eat a lot of them—don't gain weight and, in certain situations, actually lose weight? One reason for that, according to Professor Mattes, is that most nuts have a high satiety value, "meaning a person feels full after [eating] them," successfully curbing their appetite. That's one reason nutritionists have long suggested having a few nuts before you eat a meal. A second possibility is that nuts trigger an increase in an individual's resting metabolic rate, so that his or her body chemistry speeds up, burning additional energy and calories. It is also possible that people just don't chew nuts very well and only absorb a portion of their full caloric value. And finally nuts are the perfect snack food—they are filling but not crammed with sugar—and when people enjoy nuts rather than other, much more fattening snacks like potato chips, they are simply ingesting fewer calories.

There seems to be a nut for every taste, and Jessica Crandall, RDN and a well-known nutritional counselor, says, "I think they are all healthy. They are all similar in protein, fiber and fat content." However, because different nuts seem to have different nutritional value they may provide different benefits. While Crandall believes "[e]ating a variety of the different kinds will give you all of those benefits," you can choose to eat the nut or nuts that are best for you.

America's most popular nut is the peanut. Thomas Jefferson

was the first president to grow peanuts, and Jimmy Carter was the first peanut farmer to become president. Peanuts are about 30 percent protein and are packed with potassium and the B vitamins, which makes them an especially good way of avoiding cramping during workouts. The nutritional value of peanuts has been credited with enabling American agriculture to survive. By the turn of the twentieth century millions of acres of American farmland had been severely damaged by decades of growing cotton and tobacco, which robbed the soil of vital nutrients. Famed botanist George Washington Carver advised struggling farmers to rotate their crops; every other year plant peanuts and oil plants that restored minerals. Carver's advice worked, not only bringing back to life millions of acres of depleted soil but also creating a new cash crop—peanuts. In fact, Carver's plan was so successful that suddenly there was an abundance of peanuts, and he created three hundred different ways of using them.

Peanuts apparently originated in South America more than two thousand years ago. The well-known Mr. Peanut was created by a fourteen-year-old in 1916, enabling him to win the $5 grand prize in a contest sponsored by Planters Peanuts. Mr. Peanut became the Planters mascot. It is one of the most widely recognized logos in advertising history. Later, Frank P. Krize Sr. added a number of features. Mr. Peanut is now depicted in his shell, dressed as a gentleman in formal clothing, wearing a top hat, monocle, and spats and holding a cane.

One word of caution, though: All these benefits can't be gained by eating peanut butter. Peanut butter, or peanut paste, was created in 1890 by a St. Louis physician as a treat for his patients with bad teeth, and it was introduced nationally at the 1904 St. Louis World's Exposition. While peanut butter contains all of the beneficial nutrients of peanuts and in the Nurses' Health Study was equally effective in reducing the risk of cardiovascular disease, manufacturers have packed it with additional fat, sodium, and sugars, as well as hydrogenated oil to extend shelf life and maintain freshness. To gain the full benefits of peanuts from peanut butter without the inherent dangers from those additions, stick to brands that use a nonhydrogenated oil or a natural product that is made only from peanuts.

Consider the pistachio! A one-ounce serving of this cholesterol-free nut contains 10 percent of the daily requirements for fiber, magnesium, the B vitamins, copper, and phosphorus. But it is another possible benefit that has been getting attention. In a small, interesting 2011 study conducted by the Departments of 2nd Urology and Biochemistry at the Atatürk Teaching and Research Hospital in Ankara, Turkey, and published in the *International Journal of Impotence Research* in 2011, researchers gave seventeen men with high levels of LDL cholesterol who had previously complained about erectile dysfunction (ED) 100 grams of pistachio nuts every day for three weeks. Researchers speculated that the ability of pistachio nuts to reduce the risk of coronary failure by increasing blood flow might also affect other parts of the body. And in fact, they found, a "3-week pistachio diet applied to patients with ED resulted in a significant improvement in erectile function parameters . . . without any side effects."

Pistachios have the highest content of cholesterol-fighting sterol of all nuts and have been proven to help lower LDL cholesterol and fight diabetes, causing researchers at the Clinical Nutrition and Risk Factor Modification Centre at St. Michael's Hospital in Toronto to wonder if they might also affect blood sugar after a meal. In a very small study published in 2011 in the *European Journal of Nutrition,* ten people were examined after eating a meal rich in carbohydrates—both without pistachios and with the nuts added, and researchers reported the blood glucose response was dose-dependent. The more pistachios participants ate, the more the blood sugar level was reduced, causing researchers to suggest, "The beneficial effects of pistachios on post-prandial glycemia (blood sugar level after eating) could, therefore, be part of the mechanism by which nuts reduce the risk of diabetes and CHD."

Walnuts are the oldest known food to grow on trees, dating back to at least 7000 BC. The Romans knew them as "Jupiter's royal acorn" and they were so important in early trade that the world referred to them as English walnuts. In addition to a high level of omega-3 fatty acids, which are known inflammation fighters, walnuts also contain more beneficial antioxidants than any other nut. While walnuts are already shown to help fight diabetes and reduce the risk of heart disease, scientists are particularly curious about the effect of walnuts on various cancers, and in laboratory tests walnuts have demonstrated some effect on breast cancer.

Almonds are given a strong billing in the Bible; the Book of Numbers tells the story of Aaron's rod, which blossomed and bore almonds, and from then on almonds were perceived to have divine approval. They were later a prized ingredient in Egyptian breads prepared for the pharaohs. Almonds contain more fiber and more vitamin E than any other nut, which is one reason they appear to help moderate or prevent weight gain from snacking, lower the risk of type 2 diabetes, and contribute to heart health by reducing cholesterol. But they also appear to have additional benefits that, like most other nuts,

Pistachios lower LDL
cholesterol (the "bad" cholesterol)
and also offer protection against diabetes.
Each pistachio is only 4 calories.

are just being discovered. For example, a very large European epidemiological study published in 2005 in *Cancer Epidemiology Biomarkers and Prevention* by the French Nutrition and Hormones Group and supported by the International Agency for Research on Cancer and the World Health Organization examined data from almost half a million men and women and found that while eating almonds did not appear to prevent men from getting colon cancer, "a significant inverse association was observed in subgroup analyses for colon cancer in women." As in so many other studies, researchers cautioned that they had no explanation why this protection was found only in women and why it appeared to be limited to colon cancer.

Pecans are the only major tree nut that grows naturally in North America, which made it an important part of the Native American and colonial fall diet. As with most other nuts, most of the most promising research about the benefits of pecans has been done in the laboratory rather than in human studies. For example, a project at the Center for Cellular Neurobiology and Neurodegeneration Research at the University of Massachusetts showed that mice that were fed a diet supplemented with pecans showed a significant delay in the decline of motor function when compared with mice that did not eat pecans. The large amount of antioxidants found in pecans also appears to contribute to heart health; a 2011 Loma Linda University study published in the *American Journal of Nutrition* demonstrated that pecans successfully lowered LDL cholesterol by as much as 33 percent while raising important levels of vitamin E. A 2006 study conducted by the same team at Loma Linda and published by *Nutrition* showed that "adding just a handful of pecans to your diet may help inhibit unwanted oxidation of blood lipids, thus preventing coronary heart disease."

Known as "nature's vitamin pill," cashews rank among the most popular nuts in the world. Many nuts, but especially cashews, seem to be effective in reducing the risk of gallstones. More than a million American women are annually diagnosed with gallstones: hard, crystalline masses that grow in the gall bladder and can cause extreme pain and may even be fatal. An arm of the Nurses' Health Study studied the dietary practices that either led to or prevented the creation of these stones. Nuts in general proved to reduce the risk of gallstones, but women who ate cashews at least once a week saw a 25 percent reduction in their risk of developing often-debilitating gallstones.

While almost all nuts offer certain benefits, it's important to remember that some nuts actually can be dangerous; for example an estimated one hundred fifty people around the world are killed annually by falling coconuts! Coconuts are the largest nut, and a full-grown coconut can weigh as much as four and a half pounds; a coconut falling from a full-grown palm tree, which can be more than ninety feet tall, is the equivalent of about a ton of weight. But until recently, at least, most people believed that the greatest danger presented by coconuts was its oil: coconut oil was high in the type of unsaturated fats that raise cholesterol levels and lead to heart attacks. People were warned to strictly limit the amount of coconut oil they used for cooking.

But that perception is changing, and it appears that at least in some ways coconuts, as long as they don't fall on your head, actually can be beneficial. The reason is that not all coconut oils are the same. The highly processed coconut oil commonly used two decades ago contained trans fats and other dangerous, cholesterol-promoting compounds and was known for causing rapid and unhealthy spikes in cholesterol; virgin coconut oil—which was not available at that time—is the coconut oil most often used today and appears to offer a number of health benefits. In a 2009 Brazilian double-blind clinical trial published online, forty obese women ate the same diet supplemented either with healthy soy bean oil or virgin coconut oil for three months, and at the end of that time the group given coconut oil lost more weight than those women given soy bean oil. A 2013 Canadian laboratory study published in the *Journal of Alzheimer's* showed that virgin coconut oil offered some protection to the cortical neurons that are affected by Alzheimer's. And in many parts of the world coconuts have long been a staple of diets, without causing the problems usually associated with high levels of saturated fats.

So is coconut oil now considered good for you? According to Walter Willett, chairman of the Department of Nutrition at the Harvard School for Public Health, "Most of the research so far has consisted of short-term studies to examine its effect on cholesterol levels. We don't really know how coconut oil affects heart disease. And I don't think coconut oil is as healthful as vegetable oils like olive oil and soybean oil, which are mainly unsaturated fat and therefore both lower LDL and increase HDL."

While the American Heart Association continues to warn people to "[s]tay away from . . . coconut oil," it turns out that coconuts—like other nuts—happen to be a rich source of fiber, vitamins, and minerals, as well as being the source of medicines used to treat an impressive array of diseases.

While for almost everyone adding nuts to your regular diet makes good health sense, there are a few dangers that should be considered. Nut allergies, for instance, are real and poten-tially very dangerous. Approximately 1 percent of Americans suffer from nut allergies. Some children will develop immu-nity over time, but the majority will not. The best way to deal with a nut allergy is to avoid eating nuts either directly or as part of the preparation of a product. Unfortunately, that is not always as simple as it sounds. It's easy to avoid peanuts in a bowl, but chances are most people don't know when a sauce or even a shampoo contains nut oils. By law all nut products must appear on product labels, so consumers concerned about nut allergies should carefully read the label of anything they purchase. Second, anyone who has a nut allergy should always carry an epinephrine autoinjector. Epinephrine, or adrenaline, can prevent an individual from experiencing the potentially life-threatening symptoms of an allergic reaction.

So what nuts should you be eating, and how many of them is healthy for you? Personally I eat a bag of mixed nuts—cashews, pistachios, or spicy peanuts—pretty much every day. When I'm leaving the house in the morning I'll take a bag of nuts with me to eat in the car. Almost all the various types of nuts offer some health benefits, so the best thing to do is enjoy an assortment, which will provide all of those ben-efits. How much you should be eating is a matter of being sensible. Like everything else, moderation is the key. Nuts can be even more beneficial when used to replace less-healthy snack foods in your diet. A handful of nuts is substantially better for you than a chocolate sweet with artificial ingredients or a bag of chips fortified with various artificial ingredients and fats. Most studies consider a serving to be no more than two ounces; there are an estimated forty-nine pistachios in an ounce, or twenty-five almonds or seventeen macadamia nuts. Some nutritionists suggest the easiest way of adding nuts to your diet is using them to compliment other items like a tossed salad, a fish entrée, or a stir-fried dish—but probably not as an ice cream topping.

And while the mix of omega-3 fatty acids, protein, and fiber found in most nuts will make you feel satiated and reduce your appetite, it's still important to moderate your consumption.

Just as I say to my patients I offer to you this admonition, nay advice: "Go nuts!"

5

MEDITATE ONCE A
DAY—TWICE

There is a story told about a very learned man who once was asked, "What have you gained from meditation?"

The wise man shook his head and responded, "Nothing." And then he added, "But let me tell you what I lost: anger, anxiety, depression, insecurity, fear of old age and death."

While people throughout the ages have practiced meditation in one of a variety of forms for thousands of years, it appears that science has only recently discovered it. The claims made about the benefits have ranged from its simply making people feel better, healthier, and happier to its enabling them to glimpse or survive for prolonged periods in some ethereal place that exists between consciousness and the afterlife. Only recently researchers have begun seriously investigating meditation to discover if the claimed benefits are real or imagined—and more importantly, scientists are beginning to reconcile the objective physiological and neurological benefits of what had been a primarily subjective experience.

Of course, they could have just asked me.

My wife, Amita, grew up in a very spiritual home in India. Each morning her father, who was an engineer, would greet the dawn by meditating cross-legged in the lotus position on a deerskin rug. Meditation was quite common in India, and the amazing feats of the spiritual teachers, those who could control their breathing for prolonged periods of time, were well documented. As a child Amita tried to teach herself breathing techniques that promised a path to a higher level of consciousness.

My childhood was considerably less spiritual. My father was among the leading physicians in India, and my brother Deepak and I were brought up to rely on the proven techniques of Western medicine. Years later, after Deepak and I had both moved to America to practice medicine, Deepak became interested in transcendental meditation. At that time this appeared to be nothing more than a fad to me—a shortcut to enlightenment. Like so many other Americans I didn't want anything to do with it. I had had enough of it in India and associated meditation with people who wore saffron robes and walked around chanting hymns. But it did not surprise me that Amita wanted to explore it.

A month after she began meditating I noticed some distinctive changes in her; there seemed to be an aura of calm that embraced her. She looked even more beautiful, confident, and happy. Although she did not try to sell me on transcendental meditation (TM), admittedly I became curious. One Saturday morning I drove her to the local TM center in Cambridge, Massachusetts, and waited for her in the car. As I sat there reading a book about tennis there was a tap on my window. The man standing there introduced himself as Ted Weisman. I knew his name because he had taught TM to my brother.

I invited Ted to sit with me in the car and asked him to

The author has been
meditating for more than
three decades and considers
it an extraordinary gift.

tell me about TM. On the spot he gave me the introductory lecture and instantly corrected several of my misconceptions and apprehensions. I wouldn't have to give up drinking or smoking, he explained. Meditation would help me become more assertive at work, enabling me to draw strength from a strong though silent place. And most important to me at that time, it would help me become more focused and competitive when I played tennis. I happened to be in the finals of a tennis tournament and asked him whether it might help me win. He smiled and replied, "I can't guarantee that you'll win, but if you lose you won't feel so bad!"

I learned the technique of transcendental meditation the next weekend and began meditating regularly, twice a day for fifteen to thirty minutes. That was more than three decades ago, and TM continues to play an important role in my life. I consider it an extraordinary gift. I have lived the differences it makes, so none of the recent discoveries about the physical and psychological benefits that can be derived from meditation really comes as a surprise to me.

Meditation is still greatly misunderstood in the United States. While the number of people who meditate regularly has grown substantially—by some estimates more than six million people of all ages and backgrounds have learned TM—a large number of people continue to associate meditation with mystical and quasi-religious practices rather than simply accepting and appreciating its many benefits. In our incredibly fast-paced world, an environment in which our senses are continually being barraged by various stimuli in an attempt to attract and hold our attention, the concept that it is possible to slip away from all of it and go to a place of true peace and solitude, and do so without spending money, is hard to believe—unless you have already learned meditation. I recently read this concise and accurate description of meditation: "The goal of meditation isn't to control your thoughts, it's to stop letting them control you."

The claims made through the years about the benefits of meditation seem to border on the miraculous: Supposedly it reduces the need for overall medical care and cuts the occurrence of coronary events almost by half, it improves the quality of life for the aging and prolongs life, it reduces anxiety and depression and promotes intelligence and creativity, it helps you sleep better and makes you happier, and it can even help you stop smoking. Unfortunately, the quality of many of these studies was not good, and the possibility that something so easy to do and so readily accessible could make such a substantial physical and psychological impact can make meditation appear too good to be true.

But that skepticism is slowly disappearing. As the group Buffalo Springfield sang many years ago, "There's something happening here; What it is ain't exactly clear." There is no longer any doubt that meditation affects both mental and physical processes, but how it does so and exactly what it does—and how to control it and benefit from it—just isn't known. UCLA psychiatrist Dr. Rebecca Gladding wrote in *Psychology Today* in 2013, "I'm sure you've heard people extol the virtues of meditation. You may be skeptical of the claims that it helps with all aspects of life. But, the truth is, it does. Sitting every day, for at least 15–30 minutes, makes a huge difference in how you approach life, how personally you take things and how you interact with others. It enhances compassion, allows you to see things more clearly (including yourself) and creates a sense of calm and centeredness that is indescribable. There really is no substitute." There also is a growing body of scientific evidence that meditation has a real and favorable impact on a wide variety of diseases and conditions and can even make a difference in life and death.

Meditation, which might loosely be defined as a personal journey into your inner consciousness, is one of the oldest continued practices of mankind. The Hindu Vedas written about 1500 BCE report the meditative traditions of ancient India. By the sixth century BCE, different forms of meditation were developing in China and among Indian Buddhists.

By 20 BCE it had spread to the West and Philo of Alexandria wrote about "spiritual exercises" that included focused attention and concentration. Many early religious practices appear to have included some form of meditation, including Christianity and Judaism, as did developing physical systems like yoga and various martial arts. Perhaps because there has never been a single unified technique, the practice of meditation really only entered mainstream Western cultures in the 1960s, when people like the Beatles, musician Ravi Shankar, and even the commandant of the U.S. Army War College General Franklin Davis, learned TM and publicly extolled its virtues. Since then interest in various forms of meditation has skyrocketed; as Oprah Winfrey told Dr. Mehmet Oz, "The one thing I want to continue to do is to center myself every day and make that a practice for myself, because I am one thousand percent better when I do." But it is only in the last decades that science and medicine have begun exploring meditation to discover if the many reputed benefits can be proved. And while there is obviously a great deal of research to be done, there is little doubt that adding regular meditation to your life can result in substantial benefits.

Among the difficulties researchers have faced in their effort to study meditation is the fact that there are so many different forms of meditation practiced throughout the world. The National Center for Complementary and Integrative Health (NCCIH), which was founded by the NIH in 1999 to examine complementary and integrative health interventions to determine if they have any real value, defines mediation as "a mind and body practice that has a long history of use for increasing calmness and physical relaxation, improving psychological balance, coping with illness, and enhancing overall health and well-being."

While there are different kinds of meditation, according to the NCCIH most of them have four common elements: they are usually done in a quiet location with as few distractions as possible; they involve a specific, comfortable posture, usually sitting. They require people to focus their attention on any of several possibilities, including a word or words, their breathing, or even objects; and they require an open attitude, meaning distractions come and go without holding your attention. It is simply a place where your body, breath, mind, and spirit can be integrated for a brief but exquisitely beautiful period of time.

There are several different and widely followed paths to reach that mental state. These include mantra meditation, like transcendental meditation, in which a word or phrase is repeated in the mind but is not spoken out loud; relaxation response, in which a practitioner can ease his mind into a state calm; mindfulness, essentially the Buddhist concept of bringing attention to your own thoughts and surroundings, most typically focusing on your breath; and yoga and other forms that encompass breathing exercises and physical movement. There also are variations of each of these.

Meditation is easily available to everyone: It actually is quite easy to learn, costs nothing to do, can be done at your convenience in almost any environment, and appears to offer both immediate and long-term benefits. It is widely acknowledged that meditation can reduce stress and lower blood pressure, and it is well established that stress can cause several extremely serious conditions. This ability to reduce stress and lower blood pressure makes meditation a helpful tool in dealing with heart disease, anxiety, depression, anger, and hostility, and it can favorably impact insomnia. Other studies have indicated that meditation may provide some relief for people suffering a variety of different conditions ranging from irritable bowel syndrome to addictions.

Scientific evidence proving those benefits has been elusive for several reasons, among them, as Dr. Charles Raison, professor of integrative health at the University of Arizona pointed out, "A great danger in the field is that many of the researchers are also meditators, with a feeling about how powerful and useful these practices are. There has been a tendency for people to be attempting to prove what they already know."

For a long time almost all of the "evidence" we've had about the benefits of meditation has been anecdotal. Clint Eastwood, for example, said, "I'm a great supporter of Transcendental meditation. I've been using it for almost 40 years now—and I think it's a great tool for anyone to have, to be able to utilize as a tool for stress. Stress, of course, comes with almost every business. Otherwise, why would I've been doing it for all these years, for almost half of my life?" Katy Perry learned to meditate while married to Russell Brand, who credits it with helping him overcome his addictions; she told a reporter, "It's the deepest rest your brain gets. For people

Meditation is easy to do,
but it is best learned from
an experienced teacher.

that are so creative and have this kind of creative faucet that never turns off—it just continues and continues—it can be a little exhausting. My subconscious is going even when I'm sleeping. . . . So I'm never really off. And meditation is actually the one time I get to really reset." Jerry Seinfeld, who has been meditating for more than four decades, told an interviewer, "It's very hard to explain. Do you know how I was describing it to somebody? It's like having . . . you know, your phone has a charger, right? It's like having a charger for your whole body and mind. That's what Transcendental Meditation is!"

I personally have been very fortunate to lecture throughout the United States and in many countries abroad. I've written several books and been honored with a number of awards. I attribute a major part of my professional and personal success to the practice of TM twice a day for more than thirty-five years.

For many years there have been a seemingly endless series of stories told about the benefits of meditation. Typical of those many anecdotes was one told by "Buck" Montgomery, who owned the Detroit-based chemical company H. A. Montgomery. Among the efforts he took to revitalize this company in the 1980s was teaching transcendental meditation to employees. "We needed a new approach to everything," he later explained, "A new attitude, new thinking, new energy to revitalize the company and get it to take off again." Employees were encouraged to meditate for twenty minutes of company time at least once a day. The results, Montgomery said, were extraordinary: "Productivity improved dramatically. . . . Absenteeism decreased drastically, as did sick days and injuries. The

Companies whose employees
meditate have lower absenteeism
and great productivity.

creativity of our research department went up, sales increased 120% in 2 years, and profitability went up 520%."

So while there have been many similar stories of meditation improving the lives of both individuals and corporations, proving it has been a lot more difficult. And that has allowed critics to dismiss it as some form of mental hocus-pocus, perhaps nothing more than self-hypnosis or a short-lived fad. Fortunately, recent advances have made it possible to use brain-imaging technologies to record responses to meditation, providing evidence that it actually causes anatomical and functional changes in the brain. Researchers have also studied the magnitude of those changes as they relate to cognitive ability and emotions such as compassion.

Dr. Richard Davidson is an eminent neuroscientist and professor of psychology and psychiatry at the University of Wisconsin-Madison, as well as founder and chair of the Center for Investigating Healthy Minds at the Waisman Center. He has done groundbreaking research using functional MRI and electroencephalography—the latter a technique that enables him to measure electrical activity in the brain—to get a true "inside" look at the brains of people while they are meditating. He watched what happens in the brain as six monks, all of whom had been meditating for considerable periods, shifted from a state of neutral consciousness into meditation. As these monks moved into a meditative state their brains showed a very sharp transition to sustained periods of synchronized, high-amplitude oscillations in their brains' gamma frequency range. As they made the transition Davidson reported an immediate and substantial response, indicating a direct change in mental activity. A control group showed no similar response, enabling Davidson to demonstrate that meditation leads to very specific brain activity. The larger questions became, What does that mean? Is this potentially useful, and if so, how do we employ it?

In 2000 a team of researchers led by Dr. Sara Lazar, of the Department of Psychiatry at Massachusetts General Hospital and Harvard Medical School, took the next step by using an MRI to "identify and characterize the brain regions that are active during simple forms of meditation. . . . Significant signal increases were observed" in several parts of the brain. Most importantly, "The results indicate that the practice of meditation activates neural structures involved in attention and control of the autonomic nervous system." In other words, it had become possible to provide evidence that meditation results in changes in the brain. The question then became, Exactly what do the changes mean? What good does meditation do?

The results of other landmark studies have shown that regular meditation does have physiological effects that appear to provide important benefits. As reported in 2011 in the journal *Psychoneuroendocrinology,* a team of researchers from the University of California, Davis, recruited sixty people for an intensive three-month-long meditation retreat. In what was named the Shamatha project, they invited other scientists to participate by investigating different aspects of the meditators' response.

Among the participants was psychologist Elissa Epel from the University of California, San Francisco, who has been collaborating with Professor Elizabeth Blackburn. Blackburn, together with Carol Greider and Jack Szostak, received the 2009 Nobel Prize in Medicine or Physiology for her pioneering work on telomeres. Just like we have a plastic tip on the end of shoelaces, there is a cap at the end of chromosomes

Science is catching up.
Meditation leads to
impressive structural and
functional changes in the brain.

called a telomere. Shortened telomeres and decreased telo-merase activity is associated with cell aging. Individuals with shortened telomeres are at greater risk for a number of seri-ous conditions, including heart disease, diabetes, obesity, and degenerative diseases—as well as a shortened life span.

What the researchers reported was amazing. Medita-tors had "significantly greater" telomerase activity. "The data suggest," researchers concluded, "that increases in perceived control and decreases in negative activity contributed to an increase in telomerase activity, with implications for telomere length and immune cell longevity."

Dr. Epel and Dr. Blackburn joined several other research-ers in a 2004 study that demonstrated the effect of stress on telomere activity and length. This study consisted of fifty-eight mothers, half of whom were a primary caregiver for a chronically ill child. The theory that long-term stress would be reflected in telomere length proved to be accurate: "Within the caregiver group, the more years of caregiving, the shorter the mother's telomere length, the lower the telomerase activ-ity. . . ." They concluded, "Women with the highest levels of perceived stress have telomeres shorter on average by the equivalent of at least one decade of additional aging compared to low stress women." And those shorter telomeres have been associated with a variety of age-related diseases. So clearly re-ducing stress can have a profound effect on health.

It appears that many forms of meditation reduce stress. A small month-long 2012 study published in *Alternate Therapies in Health and Medicine* and conducted at the respected All In-dia Institute of Medical Sciences, in which the galvanic skin response (GSR), heart rate (HR), and salivary cortisol (a hormone release when an individual is stressed) of thirty-four

*Shortened telomerase activity
has been linked to cellular aging.
Meditators have significantly
greater telomerase activity.*

participants were measured after a stress-inducing experience, found "meditation brought significant improvements in IQ and scores for cognitive functions, whereas participants' stress levels decreased." Several other studies confirmed that meditation lessened the body's release of cortisol in stressful situations.

Another arm of the Shamatha project examined the effect of meditation on cortisol levels. "This was the first study to show a direct relation between resting cortisol and scores on any type of mindfulness [meditation] scale," according to researcher Tony Jacobs, whose results were published in *Health Psychology* in 2013. "The more a person reported directing their cognitive resources to immediate sensory experience and the task at hand, the lower their resting cortisol." In other words, the more participants were in a state of mindfulness, the lower the stress they experienced.

This reduction of stress might well be the reason that continued meditation appears to have a positive effect on long-term health. According to Dr. Raison, "We know stress is a contributor to all the major modern killers. It's hard to think of an illness in which stress and mood don't figure."

Do you know that the number one time individuals are predisposed to suffer a heart attack is Monday morning? This is a sad commentary on our lifestyle in Western countries. Many individuals are not happy at work. On Monday mornings, they are going to start a week of unhappiness and stress, often even experiencing anger on the road.

A 2009 study reported in the American Heart Association journal *Circulation* followed 201 African Americans with coronary heart disease for five years. Some of them were taught transcendental meditation, while the control group was offered health education classes. After five years researchers reported, "Stress reduction with the TM program was associated with 43% reduction in risk for all cause mortality, myocardial infarction and stroke in a high-risk sample of African Americans."

While researchers couldn't pinpoint the reasons for such a dramatic decrease, data showed that participants who meditated had lower blood pressure, considered an important risk factor for many conditions. High blood pressure, or hypertension, is known as "the silent killer"; more than sixty million Americans are at risk for dangerously high blood pressure, and it is estimated that hypertension accounts for more than twenty-five thousand deaths annually. It can severely damage many organs, among them the heart, coronary arteries, kidneys, and lungs. It is estimated that almost a third of all American adults are at risk for hypertension. A 2009 meta-analysis conducted by researchers at the University of Kentucky and published in the *American Journal of Hypertension* examined nine "randomized, controlled clinical trials that used Transcendental Meditation as a primary intervention and evaluated blood pressure changes as a primary or secondary outcome measure." This included 367 meditators and 344 in the control groups and lasted between eight and fifty-two weeks. These researchers concluded, "Transcendental Meditation is associated with a significant reduction in systolic and diastolic blood pressure of ~5 and 3 mm Hg, respectively. Sustained blood pressure reductions of this magnitude are likely to significantly reduce risk for cardiovascular disease."

Another 2009 study, conducted by the Maharishi University of Management—which emphasizes transcendental meditation—and American University, studied 298 students from

American University and other Washington, D.C., schools. Funded partially by the National Center for Complementary and Integrative Health, part of the National Institutes for Health, this randomized, controlled trial divided participants into a group that was taught TM, a control group, and a subgroup consisting of 159 people considered at high risk for hypertension based on blood pressure readings, weight, and family history. This three-month study, published in the *American Journal of Hypertension*, found overall that while blood pressure decreased in the TM group and increased in the control group, the differences were not significant—however, and perhaps most important, the differences in blood pressure within the high-risk group were significant. Researchers also reported significant improvement among all meditators compared with the control group in total psychological distress, anxiety, depression, anger or hostility, and coping ability.

In a 2014 NCCIH blind study conducted at Case University, one hundred people who were not taking any prehypertension or hypertension medications were taught mindfulness-based stress-reduction techniques as well as coping skills over an eight-week period, while the alternate arm of the study was taught progressive muscle-relaxation techniques. Participants were asked to practice these skills forty-five minutes, six days a week for eight weeks. Researchers reported in *Psychosomatic Medicine* that mindfulness-based stress reduction resulted "in substantial and statistically significant reductions in the primary outcomes." According to study author Dr. Richard Josephson, "This could prove to be an adjunct for individuals with poorly controlled blood pressure. It could also potentially decrease the need for medications as the only options for optimizing blood pressure levels."

A claim often made by proponents of meditation is that it simply makes you feel better and happier. "Feeling better" is an inexact term that is very difficult to substantiate. But when you start examining the impact of meditation on a series of psychological conditions, including anxiety and depression, it does become possible to give at least some support to those anecdotal claims. One of the largest investigations, a meta-analysis of forty-seven trials with 3,515 participants conducted by researchers at Johns Hopkins, was published in *JAMA* in 2014, "[t]o determine the efficacy of meditation programs in improving stress-related outcomes (anxiety, depression, stress/distress, positive mood, mental health–related quality of life, attention, substance use, eating habits, sleep, pain, and weight) in diverse adult clinical populations."

The results were mixed. Researchers concluded, "Mindfulness meditation programs had moderate evidence of improved anxiety at 8 weeks and at 3–6 months, depression at 8 weeks and at 3–6 months, and pain." However, they also found "low evidence of improved stress/distress and mental health-related quality of life," while pointing out that in some studies there simply was insufficient evidence to reach any determination.

While these statistical results about the effect of meditation on depression seem to be moderate at best, in fact these simple techniques have shown almost precisely the same impact on anxiety, depression, and pain as the most common antidepressant medications. As *Forbes* magazine concludes, "when it comes to treating depression, which has a notoriously low treatment success rate, the effect size for meditation in the current study is actually pretty impressive." And, as study leader Dr. Madhav Goyal pointed out, as opposed to medications that may cause other problems, "there is no known major harm from meditating, and meditation doesn't come with any known side effects. One can also practice meditation along with other treatments one is already receiving."

A 2010 meta-analysis conducted by researchers at Boston University and published in the *Journal of Consulting and Clinical Psychology* included thirty-nine studies with a total of more than a thousand participants who received mindfulness-based therapy. The premise was simply that using the techniques of mindfulness, which encourages meditators to bring all their attention to the moment, allows participants to eliminate the regrets of past events or anxieties about the future, both of which give rise to mood swings and anxiety. Researchers concluded that mindfulness-based therapy could bring significant improvements in both depression and anxiety immediately following meditation—and that these benefits persisted for several months.

Irish journalist Barry Egan once said, "Meditation made me a little bit less of a moody crankypants." While few people say it so colorfully, the most common explanation people give for why they have made meditation part of their life is simply that it makes them feel good. Scientists have tried to translate that feeling into statistical models and have conducted some interesting experiments to accomplish that. A controlled, randomized 2013 trial conducted by researchers at the University of South Carolina followed, for as long as two years, 172 women between the ages of twenty and sixty-five who had been diagnosed with early stage breast cancer, all of whom had been or were being treated with radiotherapy. A diagnosis of breast cancer almost by definition brings with it depression, anxiety, and a variety of other psychological challenges, which can make treatment much more difficult. Half of these women were enrolled in a mindfulness-based stress reduction program, while the others had nutrition education intervention. Questionnaires were used to record the responses in numerous psychosocial variables. After four months the one hundred twenty women then actively receiving radiotherapy reportedly "experienced a significant (P<.05) improvement in 16 psychosocial variables compared with the Nutrition Education-arm." Researchers concluded that meditation appeared to have real benefits as "an adjunctive therapy in oncological practice."

Dr. Sara Lazar's brain-imaging studies, conducted at Mass General and published in *Psychiatry Research: Neuroimaging* in 2011, have proved that there is a physical reason for these good feelings: "Practitioners have long claimed meditation . . . provides cognitive and psychological benefits that persist throughout the day," Lazar explained. "This study demonstrates that changes in brain structure may underlie some of these reported improvements and people are not just feeling better because they are spending time relaxing." Her group took images of the brain structure of sixteen volunteers both two weeks prior to and two weeks after they participated in a mindfulness-based stress-reduction program. According to researchers at the Mass General Hospital, "The analysis of MR images . . . found increased grey-matter density in the hippocampus, known to be important for learning and memory, and in structures associated with self-awareness, compassion and introspection. Participant-reported reductions in stress also were correlated with decreased grey-matter density in the amygdale, which is known to play an important role in anxiety and stress."

As the author of the paper, Britta Holzel, PhD, pointed

out, "It is fascinating to see . . . that by practicing meditation we can play an active role in changing the brain and can increase our well being and quality of life."

This ability to reduce stress has been shown to provide real benefits for people fighting several serious diseases. In addition to ongoing studies about the ability to prevent disease or modify the severity, there is evidence that meditation can be an important tool in managing a disease. A randomized, controlled 2000 study conducted at the Baker Cancer Centre in Alberta, Canada, and published in *Psychosomatic Medicine*, divided ninety-one patients diagnosed with a variety of different cancers at different stages into a group that was taught mindfulness and meditated regularly for seven weeks and a wait-listed group that did not. The results were impressive. Researchers reported, "Patients in the treatment group had significantly lower scores on Total Mood Disturbance, and subscales of Depression, Anger, Anxiety and Confusion and more Vigor than control subjects. The treatment group also had fewer overall symptoms of stress, fewer Cardiopulmonary and gastrointestinal symptoms, less emotional irritability, Depression and Cognitive Disorganization, and fewer habitual patterns of stress. Overall reduction in Total Mood Disturbance was 65% with a 31% reduction in symptoms of stress."

At the conclusion of the initial program those patients on the waiting list were taught the same meditative techniques and after completion reported the same response. According to study author Linda Carlson, PhD, "At the time of diagnosis, patients felt isolated, scared and unsure of what to do. The MBCR program helped them to feel less isolated in their journey. It taught concrete tools for self-regulation and introduced new ways to look at the world. For them, this

Meditators change their brain ("neuroplasticity") and have a feeling of well-being as well as a greater ability to handle stressful events.

resulted in fewer stress symptoms and lower levels of mood disturbance."

This was one of the studies the American Cancer Society referred to when it advised that "available scientific evidence does not suggest that meditation is effective in treating cancer or any other disease; however, it may help to improve the quality of life for people with cancer," adding that "[r]esearch shows that meditation can help reduce anxiety, stress, blood pressure, chronic pain, and insomnia" and that "[m]ost experts agree that the positive effects of meditation outweigh any negative reactions."

Another common medical condition that experts agree is exacerbated by stress is irritable bowel syndrome, a chronic disorder of the lower gastrointestinal tract that can result in pain, gas, diarrhea, or constipation and for which there is no cure. As reported in the *American Journal of Gastroenterology* in 2011, researchers at the University of North Carolina's School of Medicine wondered if it was possible to reduce symptoms by teaching patients the stress-reducing techniques in meditation. They randomly assigned seventy-five female patients into two groups, teaching one group mindfulness meditation and the other group traditional strategies for dealing IBS. The results were impressive: Immediately after the eight-week trial those women using mindfulness showed a 26.4% reduction in the severity of symptoms while the control group reported only a 6.2% reduction. Far more impressive were the results after three months, at which time meditators reported a 38.2% reduction while the control group showed only an 11.8% reduction. The researchers concluded, "Mindfulness training has a substantial therapeutic effect on irritable bowel severity, improves health related quality-of-life and reduces stress."

A similar 2013 randomized, ninety-patient study conducted at the University of Calgary and published in the *International Journal of Behavioral Medicine* concluded that IBS patients who received mindfulness-based, stress-reduction training showed improvement that was clinically meaningful, with symptom severity decreasing from constant to occasionally present . . . At six month follow-up the MBSR group maintained a clinically meaningful improvement in IBS symptoms compared to the wait-list group."

Dr. Holzel added, "Other studies . . . have shown that meditation can make significant improvements in a variety of symptoms." And while there has not been a significant amount of good research done concerning the value of meditation to fight specific diseases and behaviors, the research that has taken place has shown interesting but mixed results for several different conditions—including hard-to-break habits and addictions.

Mark Twain once quipped that stopping smoking was one of the easiest things he had ever done; in fact, it was so easy he did it seven or eight times! The reality is that smoking is a very difficult habit to break, but there has been considerable evidence that meditation can be helpful in breaking this habit. In a small 2013 study done at the University of Oregon and published online in the *Proceedings of the National Academy of Sciences,* researchers recruited twenty-seven smokers who averaged ten cigarettes day—and who were not told the actual purpose of the study. Instead they were told researchers wanted to evaluate the effects of meditation on stress and performance. Fifteen participants were taught the techniques of mindfulness meditation, and after two weeks they had reduced their smoking by 60%, while those in the control group had not changed their behavior. More than a month later five people who had learned meditation reported they continued their changed behavior. Texas Tech researcher Yi-Yuan Tang, a coauthor of the study, suggested, "Because mindfulness meditation promotes personal control and has been shown to positively affect attention and an openness to internal and external experiences, we believe that meditation may be helpful for coping with symptoms of addiction."

A study done by Yale University's Department of Psychiatry in 2011 compared the value of meditation with the American Lung Association's Freedom from Smoking (FFS) program. Eighty-eight smokers were randomly assigned toeither a meditation program or the FFS program and met twice weekly for four weeks. At the end of that period, as reported in the journal *Drug and Alcohol Dependence*, "Compared to those randomized to the FFS intervention, individuals who received Mindfulness training showed a greater rate of reduction in cigarette use during treatment and maintained these gains during follow-up." In fact, seventeen weeks after the conclusion of this study, 31% of meditators had stopped or reduced their smoking, while only 6% of those assigned to the intervention had done so. Although about a third may not seem like a substantial number, in smoking-cessation programs it is considered a very high success rate.

It would not be accurate to claim that meditation is a proven strategy for stopping smoking or, for that matter, for changing a whole range of behaviors. While for the first time respected investigators are seriously trying to understand the benefits of meditation, about all that can be said is certain forms of meditation appear to make it easier for a sizeable number of people to change undesirable behaviors. In 2013, the Department of Neurology at Oregon's Health and Science University conducted a meta-analysis of qualified studies investigating the role meditation can play in stopping smoking. These researchers, also reporting in *Drug and Alcohol Dependence,* found that only fourteen clinical trials of the efficacy of mind-body practices to aid smoking cessation met their criteria and concluded that those studies "support yoga and meditation-based therapies as candidates to assist smoking cessation." However, researchers added, more studies needed to be done.

Certainly the results have been intriguing, although it continues to be difficult to measure the effect of a neurological process in changing ingrained physical habits. A very small 2008 study at the University of Wisconsin included fifteen alcohol-dependent adults who had completed an intensive outpatient program. Reporting in the *Journal of Addiction Medicine*, researchers found that about half of the participants were able to remain abstinent and described meditation as a "very important . . . useful relapse prevention tool" and that they were "very likely to continue meditating." The volunteers reported that the "most valuable aspects" of meditation-related training included "gaining skills to reduce stress," "real-life skills for coping with craving," and "group support."

In addition to the impact meditation appears to make on dealing with disease and conditions, it also seems to have an impact on aspects of life that aren't easily defined by statistics, among them concentration, interpersonal relationships, and optimism. There have been several studies demonstrating the value of meditation in both school and the workplace. Typical of those studies was one conducted by researchers at the

University of California, Santa Barbara, and published in *Psychological Science* in 2013. In this study twenty-four undergraduate students were randomly assigned to take a course in mindful meditation that emphasized the physical posture and mental strategies of focused-attention meditation, while a second group of twenty-four students were given a nutrition course. These courses met four times a week for forty-five minutes for two weeks. Each student took the Graduate Record Examination both before beginning and after completing the courses, as well as distractibility and memory tests. After those classes concluded, the average score of the meditation group on the GRE verbal reasoning exam increased from 460 to 520, and the group also improved on the focus and working memory tests, whereas the nutrition group showed no improvement. The lead author of the study, Michael Mrazek, attributed the gain to an increased ability to concentrate, explaining, "What surprised me the most was actually the clarity of the results. . . . This is the most complete and rigorous demonstration that mindfulness can reduce mind-wandering, one of the clearest demonstrations that mindfulness can improve working memory and reading, and the first study to tie all this together to show that mind-wandering mediates the improvements in performance,"

Those benefits seem to be equally applicable to the workplace. A 2012 study at the University of Washington, supported by the MacArthur Foundation and the National Science Foundation, investigated the ability of meditation to make multitasking in the office more productive. Researchers recruited forty-five female human resource managers and assigned them to three groups: Group A received eight weeks of mindfulness meditation training, Group B was the control group and was given no training, and Group C was given training in body relaxation techniques. At the beginning of the study, to establish a baseline, all participants were tested for various aspects of multitasking, which included speed and accuracy, while performing typical office tasks like word processing, sending e-mails, creating calendars, and instant messaging. The test areas were identified as "overall test time," "number of activities," and "time per activity." After training the tests were repeated, and researchers reported, "Those in the meditation group (but not in the other two groups) showed greater time on task and a reduced number of task switches as compared with pre-training and the meditators showed improved memory for the work they were doing (as did those in the relaxation group)," allowing them to conclude, "Meditation training may effect positive changes in the multitasking practices of computer-based knowledge workers."

People often ask if children and adolescents can learn and benefit from TM. There is no question that stress is encountered by young people at school, in social encounters, and even at home. Stressed kids are vulnerable to depression and anxiety and have a greater propensity to use addictive drugs. TM is easy and effortless and does not require concentration. Kids don't have to sit perfectly still. Recent estimates suggest that more than 150,000 children worldwide have learned TM. Children as young as ten years old can be instructed in this technique. They are taught to practice it for ten minutes twice a day. Many children I know do meditation with their siblings or their parents.

Certainly one of the most dramatic examples of the potential of meditation to change overall behavior is the story of San Francisco's Visitacion Valley Middle School. In 2007 this was a very rough school. Situated in one of the city's poorest neighborhoods, about 90 percent of its students came from disadvantaged environments, and about 40 percent required remedial English-language instruction. Discipline in the school had nearly broken down; attendance was spotty, and there was a high percentage of dropouts, suspensions, and fights. But that year the school began experimenting with what was called quiet time, fifteen-minute periods in the morning and afternoon when the entire school, both the faculty and the students, could either sit quietly or meditate. According to the principal, James Dierke, "We were looking for a way to get kids to relax. We saw kids with real post-traumatic stress disorder symptoms. I noticed a lot of them missing school, fighting, and getting angry a lot. They couldn't concentrate on school." The results were impressive: Since starting the program there has been a 65 percent reduction in truancy, a 50 percent reduction in suspensions, and a 0.5 percent school-wide improvement in grade point average.

As one eighth-grade student explained, "It takes away the anger. Your brain is like a lake holding in water, and when we meditate, the flood gates open and the water is released." Dierke himself stated flatly, "It's working. It is nourishing these children and providing them an immensely valuable tool for life. It is saving lives."

Other schools saw the results and instituted similar programs. Nearby Burton High School, for example, saw a 75 percent decrease in suspensions and a rise in academic performance. Three thousand miles away the small New Haven New Horizons (High) School instituted a daily transcendental meditation program and its results have been equally dramatic. "It's incredible," said Diana Gregory, a math teacher.

"The disposition of the students has changed. They're inter-ested in school; they're happy. . . . That aggression is gone." One of her students, she added, has gone from an F in algebra to an A, "[a]nd the only difference is TM."

Many of these quiet-time programs have been sponsored by the David Lynch Foundation, which has set out to offer TM to students as a means to increase academic performance while reducing stress and violence. After teaching the tech-niques of TM to 150,000 students the foundation reports that high school graduation rates have increased by 15 percent, college and postsecondary acceptances have increased by 18 percent, and there ahas been an average of double-digit improvements in GPA and test scores and a decrease in de-pression, violence, substance abuse, and suspensions.

David Lynch, in his book *Catching the Big Fish,* likens his first experience with TM to cutting an elevator cable and falling into bliss. "When I had my first mediation, this inner bliss revealed itself so powerfully—thick happiness came rush-ing in and I said, 'This is it.' There it was. And everything just started getting better—way more fun, way more joy in the doing. Everything just got better and better. I didn't think about not getting angry—the anger just lifted away. And what they say is when you start infusing this transcendence, you don't really realize that anger is going. It's other people close to you that see it first. And it just seems natural. You're happy, and there's nothing you can do about it. You just get happier."

My own experience has been very similar. When I first learned TM and I would be at a traffic intersection, I would find that people in adjacent cars were smiling at me. Initially I was confused, until I realized I was so much happier and

In schools where children are struggling, an innovative intervention—practicing meditation—leads to significant reduction in suspensions and improved academic performance.

had a big grin on my face. They were simply reacting to my bliss.

Corporations, among them giants like Apple and Google, are increasingly making meditation programs available to employees, many of them providing both time and a quiet place for those employees to simply shed workday stress. General Mills, for example, has infused its corporate culture with mindful meditation. The insurance giant Aetna has done the same thing, resulting, according to its CEO, in a 7 percent reduction in its corporate health-care costs.

Perhaps the most ubiquitous claim made by proponents of meditation is that it simply makes you feel good. It increases an individual's overall sense of well-being and happiness. As ABC News reported in 2011, "Several studies suggest that . . . meditation can make you happier, less stressed—even nicer to other people." In a study they cite, Emory University professor Chuck Raison, who recorded numerous people over a period of time, some of whom had been taught meditation and an equal number who had not, found the meditators were "more empathic with other people. They were spending more time with other people, they laughed more. They didn't use the 'I' word as much as they used the word 'we.'"

Psychology Today strongly recommended meditation in a 2013 article, "20 Scientific Reasons to Start Meditating," that enumerated the scientific reasons it improved daily life. Among those reasons, each of them supported by studies, are the following: "It 'Boosts Your Happiness' by increasing positive emotion while decreasing depression, anxiety and stress. It 'Boosts Your Social Life' by making you more compassionate, less lonely and increasing social interactions. It 'Boosts

Your Self-Control' and 'Improves Productivity' and even 'Makes You Wiser.' "

Among the many misconceptions that prevent people from investigating meditation, perhaps the major one is that it is a religion or is part of a religion or has some religious connection. It doesn't, in any sense. While there are religions that do include periods of meditative contemplation, meditation is a stand-alone practice. It has no connection to any religious practice. There are people who associate meditation and prayer, but the two practices are very different, although prayer might also lead to deep thought and relaxation. I know a Catholic priest and a rabbi who have both practiced TM for years and have said that it brought them clarity and a greater appreciation of their own sacred religion. Of course, I also know agnostics and atheists who are happily practicing TM.

There also are many people who believe meditation involves sitting rigidly in the lotus position or investing long periods of time or having to be in a specific and quiet place—absolutely none of which is true. Most forms of meditation suggest people limit their sessions to no more than twenty minutes at a time, and while it is recommended that it be done in a quiet place, that isn't necessary. It is recommended meditators sit comfortably in any position, and it can be done pretty much anywhere. There are people, for example, who meditate on the New York City subway system during their daily commute. Meditation is supposed to fit into your day and make you more productive rather than interrupt the day and make you feel guilty if you miss a day.

Some people believe that meditation is too difficult for them to learn or that it costs too much, but neither is true.

While one can learn meditation from books or on the Internet, it is best to learn it from a bona fide teacher. And finally, unlike almost anything else you might do to improve your health and your life, there is no potential downside to meditation. The worst meditation can do for anyone is nothing; one simply won't feel any of the many potential benefits. But the vast majority of people who meditate claim to have experienced at least some benefit. And I'm one of them: For me, meditation is the best thing I have done in the last three decades, and I attribute a lot of my success in all the areas of my life to the regular practice of transcendental meditation. It's only recently that science has been able to prove—by mapping changes in the brain during meditation—that those feelings that I have experienced have a physiological basis. When I learned to meditate, few of the benefits were known. Since then there have been numerous good studies demonstrating the benefits of meditation in all parts of our lives.

I treasure the twenty to thirty minutes of TM that I do in the morning and the fifteen to twenty minutes I do most evenings. While I really enjoy the feeling of peace and glow that I experience while meditating, the main reason I and others do it is to accrue the benefits in activity.

Let me leave you with an ancient aphorism: You should meditate once a day, and if you don't have time to do that, you should meditate twice a day.

CONCLUSION:
CLOSE CALLS

Many thousands of scientists and researchers go to work every day trying to solve the endlessly fascinating mysteries of the human body. Why does vitamin D seem to have the effect on good health that it does? What types of exercise provide the greatest benefit? Peanuts or walnuts? But while we know for certain that the five things recommended in this book will have actual and lasting benefits, there certainly are many other things you can try that have proven to provide real benefits. But we haven't included them because, unlike the five things we recommend heartily here, for some people there may be some serious side effects that need to be considered before adapting such measures, such as adding aspirin or dieting to your health regimen.

For several decades aspirin was the friendly pain and headache remedy. It was available at every pharmacy and everyone kept it in their medicine chest or carried it with them. It was great for all the minor aches and pains. But that all changed in 1989 when the *New England Journal of Medicine* reported that friendly old aspirin reduced the risk of a first heart attack in men by an astonishing 44 percent. The landmark Physicians'

Health Study was a randomized, double-blind, placebo-controlled national trial conducted to determine the impact of a daily aspirin on cardiovascular disease. The study included 22,071 male physicians, and the results were so conclusive that the study was stopped years ahead of schedule and the FDA recommend the use of aspirin for the prevention of heart attacks.

In fact, there has been such a wealth of evidence demonstrating the benefits of aspirin in preventing heart attacks and strokes that I advise my patients—and my friends—to carry aspirin with them at all times. You should keep it at home, in your car, in your purse or briefcase, and in your office. Keep it handy; it can save your life. The moment you feel crushing chest pains, chew an aspirin and call 911; if the pain is not a sign of a heart problem, it will likely cause no serious problems. But if it is heart related it will thin your blood, helping to maintain blood flow to your heart, and provide the extra time you may need to get medical assistance.

Aspirin may well be the oldest drug in continuous use in history. The Egyptians reportedly were using it to relieve back pain by 1500 BCE. Hippocrates wrote sometime around 400 BCE that a powder made from the bark and leaves of the willow tree would alleviate headaches, fevers, and other common ailments. In the mid-1800s it was chemically modified to make it more palatable, creating the acetylsalicylic acid we know as aspirin today. At the turn of the twentieth century German chemist Felix Hoffman named it aspirin, the "a" for the buffering content, "spir" from the plant *Spiraea ulmaria* from which it is extracted, and the suffix "in," which is commonly used in medicines. Aspirin rapidly became the most commonly used remedy in the world. But until 1989 few people realized how potentially potent aspirin actually might be. Because the legal protection for aspirin had expired decades earlier no one company owned the patent. It is inexpensive to produce and many different companies market their own aspirin. But because there is no way to protect an aspirin patent companies were not willing to invest in studies to determine its benefits—or, in some cases, its dangers.

When the results of the 1989 study were announced, researchers in academia began wondering if this "wonder drug" might have additional previously unknown benefits. They began pouring over data collected in various studies for many years. And what they found was astonishing. It was as if the demur young woman had taken off her glasses, let down her hair, and revealed herself to be a beautiful lady. Suddenly researchers began looking at the common aspirin in uncommon ways—and what they found was truly amazing. Aspirin has turned out to be the little medicine that could. In addition to preventing initial heart attacks, aspirin has been shown in clinical studies to have many other benefits. The British Doctors' Aspirin Study, for example, reported that people who had taken regular 300 milligrams of aspirin daily for five years reduced the risk of colon cancer by 74 percent over the next ten to fifteen years. Several subsequent studies confirmed that strong association. Not only that, a Massachusetts General Hospital and Harvard Medical School study reported in the *Journal of the American Medical Association* in 2009 that aspirin also reduced mortality in people diagnosed with localized colorectal cancer by between a third and a half, depending on how long they have been talking it.

In other studies aspirin has been shown to play a preventive role in a variety of other cancers. For example, the *Journal of Lower Genital Tract Disease* reported a study done at Roswell Park Cancer Institute that matched 328 patients with cervical cancer to more than a thousand controls to show that women who took an aspirin daily for more than five years lowered their risk of being diagnosed with cervical cancer by 47 percent. A 2015 meta-analysis conducted by researchers at the Duke University School of Medicine using data from 6,390 patients with an elevated PSA found that men who regularly took aspirin or other nonsteroidal anti-inflammatory drugs were 13 percent less likely to be diagnosed with prostate cancer. Other studies have shown that it reduces the chance of being diagnosed with stomach or esophageal cancers. In summation, in a 2012 study published in the respected British journal the *Lancet*, researchers at the University of Oxford analyzed fifty-one studies in which a group that took an aspirin every day was compared with a group that took no aspirin. Researchers reported that people who had taken a low-dose aspirin daily for a minimum of three years reduced their likelihood of being diagnosed with any form of cancer by 25 percent. A daily low-dose aspirin also reduced chances that an existing cancer would metastasize and begin spreading.

With strong evidence to indicate that this inexpensive tablet or pill can work wonders, shouldn't everyone be taking a low-dose aspirin every day? In fact, many doctors actually began recommending to their patients that they take a low dose—81 milligrams, or "baby aspirin"—every day as a preventive measure.

But aspirin can be very dangerous; it is not benign. As an old advertising slogan once promised, aspirin can work wonders—but it also can wreak havoc on your system. The anti-inflammatory properties of aspirin, its ability to increase blood flow by preventing platelets from clumping, which is believed to be the reason it is so successful in preventing heart attacks, may also be the reason it can be very dangerous. Preventing those clumps makes it more difficult to stop bleeding, and the regular use of aspirin has been found—in some people—to promote serious episodes. As the *British Medical Journal* reported in 2012, "the risks of aspirin outweigh its benefits in people without cardiovascular disease." According to researchers, even a low-dose aspirin taken regularly can cause or exacerbate gastric ulcers, and if people do start bleeding it will be difficult to stem the flow. Also, patients that have a stroke are more likely to experience severe bleeding, and patients who suffer any type of trauma have an increased likelihood of severe bleeding.

Additionally, regular aspirin use can damage the lining of your gastrointestinal tract, increasing the risk for a variety of serious problems, including duodenal ulcers, inflammatory bowel disease, and even Crohn's disease.

Dr. Christopher Cannon, a cardiologist at Brigham and Women's Hospital and professor of medicine at Harvard Medical School, cautions, "A lot of people take aspirin who really shouldn't. Everyone assumes aspirin is harmless, but it isn't."

Dr. Alison Bailey, director of the cardiac rehabilitation program at the University of Kentucky's Gill Heart Institute, warned of potential dangers when she told a reporter, "I stop a lot more people taking aspirin than I start. People don't even consider aspirin a medicine, or consider that you can have side effects from it. That's the most challenging part of aspirin therapy."

Cardiologists at Baylor University School of Medicine analyzed the records of seventy thousand patients using aspirin to prevent heart attacks, and in 2015 reported that 12 percent of those people did not need the aspirin and were putting themselves at risk for gastrointestinal bleeding and brain bleeds, which area type of stroke.

In an effort to determine the value of aspirin to prevent a heart attack, researchers at London's St. George University analyzed data from nine randomized studies that included more than one hundred thousand participants. Their results, published in 2012 in the *Annals of Internal Medicine*, showed that the regular users of aspirin reduced chances of suffering a heart attack by 10 percent—but also were 30 percent more likely to suffer serious gastrointestinal bleeding. In fact, for every nonfatal heart attack it prevented, aspirin caused two serious bleeding events. Dr. Sreenivasa Seshasai of St. George's Cardiovascular Sciences Research Centre said, "We have been able to show quite convincingly that in people without a previous heart attack or stroke, regular use of aspirin may be more harmful than it is beneficial."

For a long time the potential dangers of aspirin were lost in the euphoria about its many benefits. But in 2014 the FDA, which had been promoting that daily little pill for more than a decade, reassessed that position, warning, "The FDA has concluded that the data do not support the use of aspirin as a preventive medication by people who have not had a heart attack, stroke or cardiovascular problems, a use that is called 'primary prevention.' In such people the benefit has not been established but risks, such as dangerous bleeding into the brain or stomach—are still present."

So who should be taking a daily low-dose aspirin? The answer is nobody should be doing so without first discussing it with a physician. Like any other drug, aspirin can react with other things that you're taking—especially strong blood thinners. That doesn't mean you shouldn't take aspirin, but rather you should make certain your physician is aware of it so he or she can advise you appropriately.

Those people for whom a low-dose aspirin a day is recommended include people who have already had a heart attack or stroke; who have had a stent implanted in an artery; who have had coronary bypass surgery; who are at a high risk of having a heart attack, factoring in known contributing factors like family history, being overweight, and personal habits; and men over fifty and women over sixty who have diabetes and at least one other heart disease risk factor, including diabetes and high cholesterol.

Conversely, people who have chronic liver and kidney disease or have three or more alcoholic drinks a day or are known to be allergic to aspirin definitely should not be taking a daily dose. People with high blood pressure should avoid aspirin until they are able to lower their blood pressure.

Let me emphasize again that aspirin is a minor miracle and for millions of people contributes to good health—but it is not risk free and no one should be taking an aspirin regularly without consulting a physician.

The second close call was your diet. There is no question that a healthy diet will contribute to good health, the only question is what is a healthy diet? The answer is that one man's fish is another man's *le poisson*. Each of us responds to those foods we eat in very different ways and what is good for one person may not necessarily be healthy for another. Actually the word "dieting" is used broadly to describe both a temporary change in your eating habits with the objective of losing weight or an entirely new way of choosing foods for the rest of your life.

Diets work. People who strictly follow a diet will lose some weight over some period of time. There are numerous different types of diets and some of them simply are not healthy. These fad diets encourage people to stop eating certain foods or eat only other foods. The Harvard School of Public Health and Pennington Biomedical Research Center in Baton Rouge randomly assigned eight hundred overweight people to one of four heart-healthy popular diets. They included two low-fat diets that derived 20 percent of calories from fat and two high-fat diets with 40 percent of calories from fat. Participants also were encouraged to exercise at least ninety minutes a week and were given regular weight-loss counseling. After six months, across all four diet groups, the average weight loss was thirteen pounds. After two years all dieters had lost nine pounds and between one and three inches from their waist.

The evidence is that there are many, many diets that work. The more difficult problem is sustaining that weight loss for a long time. As UCLA professor Traci Mann reported in a meta-analysis of thirty-one dieting studies, published in 2007 in *American Psychologist*, "We found that the majority of people regained all the weight, plus more. . . . Diets do not lead to sustained weight loss or health benefits for the majority of people."

Other people make permanent lifestyle changes, following sensible diets associated with proven health benefits. Currently among the most popular lifestyle diets are the Paleo diet, which consists essentially of foods that cavemen might have eaten, like meats and berries, but excludes things they would not have had access to, like dairy products, and the Mediterranean diet, which emphasizes plant-based foods, including fruits and vegetables, grains and nuts, and using additives like olive oil, herbs, and spices rather than butter and salt. Both of these diets come from different parts of the world and are based on the fact that people who traditionally ate those foods lived long and healthy lives.

The Mediterranean diet has been especially popular for at least two decades. Researchers first became interested in it when they noted that people who lived in areas near the Mediterranean Sea seemingly had lower rates of cardiovascular disease and heart disease—even those people who smoked regularly—than residents of other industrialized nations. There have been many studies to try to determine the reasons for that. In one of the largest studies, researchers in the Department of Medical and Surgical Care at the University of Florence conducted a meta-analysis of the benefits of adhering to the Mediterranean diet. This included nineteen studies that ranged in time from four to twenty years and included 2,190,627 subjects. The results, published in 2010 in the *American Journal of Clinical Nutrition*, found that people who followed this diet had lower overall mortality rates, as well as reduced chances of being diagnosed with a serious disease, including heart disease, stroke, cancer, and Alzheimer's Disease. Other studies have shown a variety of benefits that include reducing the incidence of heart attack by as much as 25 percent.

The Mediterranean diet will work for some people for some time. But among several issues with it is that it includes a substantial amount of olive oil, which consists of 14 percent saturated fat and is certainly not considered a health food, and fish, which can contain mercury, so its intake should be limited. It also is not an especially cost-effective diet, as the ingredients can be expensive. It's also important to remember that this diet was created hundreds of years ago by people who often worked in the fields, walked miles every day, and did not have access to other choices.

The Paleo diet, also known as the caveman diet, was developed by a researcher at Colorado State University, who believes that these are the foods that humans were genetically designed to eat several thousand years ago. It's an interesting theory, but as researchers from Kent State and Georgia State University wrote in the *Quarterly Review of Biology* in 2014, there is no such thing as a Paleo diet. Cavemen ate whatever was available to them in the area in which they lived. Cavemen who lived in the northern latitudes were more dependent on meat, while those in the more temperate regions probably had a plant-based diet. The Paleo diet does not include any grains or dairy, both of which eaten in moderation can be beneficial, and it might not be healthy to eliminate them completely from your diet.

A vegan diet, which does not include any animal products, has been shown to have seminal health benefits. Among the chief proponents of this is the legendary Dr. Dean Ornish, a pioneer in the field of nutrition and health. His diet has been shown to actually reverse coronary heart disease, decrease angiogenesis and even have an effect on early cancers.

The very best way to lose weight is to simply eat less and exercise more. There are potential benefits but some real dangers involved in following any diet. The reality is each of us is unique and we all have our own needs and dangers. Popular diets today are designed and marketed for profit. That

doesn't mean they aren't good, just that they have been created to appeal to a large number of people and within that
group there inevitably will be many people who respond differently to the diet. Their bodies may need certain things not
part of that particular diet, proteins for instance in some diets, starch in others.

The reason any particular diet is not among the recommendations in this book is that there is a lack of uniformity
and a great lack of real scientific evidence that any of them
work to reduce weight or contribute to a healthy lifestyle—
for everyone. An interesting study conducted by researchers
at Stanford University and published in *JAMA* in March 2007
randomly assigned three hundred overweight or obese pre-
menopausal women to one of four popular diets: the low-carb
Atkins, the moderate-carb Zone diet, the low-fat LEARN
(lifestyle, exercise, attitudes, relationships, and nutrition) diet,
and the very low-fat Dean Ornish diet, which was designed
specifically to prevent or combat heart disease. After a year
the women in the Atkins group had lost an average of ten
pounds, while the three other groups averaged between four
and five pounds lost. Those in the Atkins group also saw beneficial drops in cholesterol and blood pressure. But some participants in all groups lost as much as thirty pounds. While
that result would argue for the Atkins diet, there remains considerable debate about its overall safety. Low-carb diets generally have reduced nutritional value, and people on the Atkins
diet have reported a range of problems serious enough that
the American Heart Association specifically does not recommend it.

A healthy diet can make an enormous difference to your
well-being. It is well known what foods are generally healthy

and what foods can cause problems. Eating healthy can be equated to eating sensibly: Eat reasonable portions of a variety of foods, being sure to include some protein, grains, and fat with each meal. Cut down on sugary snacks, including chips and soft drinks. Eat three meals daily and cut down considerably on snacks. Determine your personal food profile—which foods leave you feeling full and groggy and which provide energy. What are you eating too much of? Bread and grains? Dairy treats? Candy and sweets? Can you cut back on them without feel deprived?

The best thing to do is consume three regular meals a day, starting with a healthy breakfast. Find a diet program that fits your lifestyle and allows you to eat those foods you can't live without. Find a time to include exercise, drink some coffee, and add some nuts between meals.

The list of those things that have proved to be good for you is a long one. It includes things like alcohol, statins, and different types of integrative medicine. But each of them, like aspirin and diet, also can be dangerous in certain situations.

Your health is in good hands—your own: "Your diet is a bank account. Good food choices are a good investment." Bethenny Frankel

ACKNOWLEDGMENTS

Dr. Chopra and I were quite fortunate to have the assistance of many people as we worked on this book. While we would like to offer our appreciation to all of them, there are several people whose help must be acknowledged: First, our editor, Will Anderson, who was continually encouraging and enthusiastic—and always with good cheer. Our publisher, Tom Dunne, helped conceive this book and has been supportive every day. Editor Peter Joseph, whose endless hours of work on our first book certainly made this journey easier. On this book, and others, our work was greatly assisted by the writer and researcher's friend, the best transcription service I've encountered, Cass Masters' Scribecorps. My lifelong friend Jerry Stern knows how much I appreciate his contribution, as does my mostly wise friend Richard Soll. And finally, my family: my wife, Laura, the finest personal trainer and yoga instructor in New York, whose passion for health and fitness guided me; our sons, Taylor and Beau; and our dog with the heart of gold, Willie/Willow.

—*David Fisher*

Acknowledgments

I am grateful to David Fisher for our enduring friendship and collaboration. I thank Will Anderson for his support and encouragement. Heartfelt gratitude to Tom Dunne, our publisher, for his advice and wisdom over the years, and to Peter Joseph for his steadfast help in myriad ways.

—*Sanjiv Chopra*

INDEX